Birth ROCKS

Dedications

This book is dedicated to any woman who has ever been frightened of giving birth. May this book guide you towards optimism and self-awareness.

I would like to thank my amazing husband Mike and the small bundle of joy that is my son Caelen for their support, patience and cuddles.

Love and light to all of the amazing ladies at YogaBellies who live the dream of supporting women during this most important time of their lives, every single day.

Special thanks to the beautiful women who have shared their birth stories to help guide you towards your own unique birth.

Contents

Introduction: About Me

The purpose of this book is to approach the topic of pregnancy and birth with honesty, but also with optimism. I've read lots of books and seen lots of films about child birth that promised me pain free and even orgasmic births. This book is not one of them.

I'd like to caveat that by saying that I wholeheartedly believe that the day I gave birth to my son was the most amazing day of my life. And I also believe that it can be the most amazing day of your life too. I'm sure you've picked up this book hoping to find out something about childbirth that is going to help you feel more confident, knowledgeable and empowered to be able to give birth and I hope that this is what you find here.

I'm not going to provide you with a list of drugs or interventions (although we will talk about them as an option you may want to consider) and I'm not going to flummox you with extensive medical terminology either. I don't want to preach to you about why you must have a natural birth or in fact, preach to you at all (boring!)

I am writing this to book to reassure you that every single woman on this planet is entitled to the most amazing birth experience possible. I'd like to explain why we are so scared of giving birth and why we really shouldn't be scared, but looking forward to the experience. I will happily share my personal experience of pregnancy and birth and also share with you, the birth stories of other women from across the world who wants to reach out and reassure you too. You are going to give birth the same way that millions of women over millions of year of human history have given birth before you. Giving birth is the most beautiful, unique experience a woman will ever have.

Before I get carried away, I want to tell you a little bit about me. I want you to be able to get to know and trust yourself and to be completely honest with yourself, and so it's probably best to start with me. Another thing I want you to know about me, is that I am just your average mother of one.

I am 33 years old, a yoga teacher and antenatal educator and happily married mother of one adorable little man. I was a business analyst and a marketing manager in a past life and when I was made redundant during pregnancy, I founded YogaBellies and Birth ROCKS. I have now worked with hundreds of pregnant and new mothers and train perinatal yoga teachers and birth mentors across the world, which I love.

Although I have practised and taught yoga for many years, I have never spent time in the mountains, consuming only goji berries and drinking only mountain dew. I have sadly, never even been to India where many of the great teachers study. I have no special 'magikal' powers and my pain threshold is pretty low (yes, I cry when I stand on lego too.) I watch Eastenders and I probably drink more diet coke than is good for me. The point is that I am no more 'qualified' than any other woman to give birth and I had an amazing birth experience.

You don't need to be a yoga teacher or a Spiritual Goddess, you just need to know and understand yourself before you go into birth. Every woman is entitled to a beautiful birth and I'd like to help you to have that experience. I'll explain a little more by telling you about my journey.

I was first introduced to yoga by a handsome young Swedish student in my first year at University. We used to stand on our heads and chant, although not necessarily in that order. The relationship didn't last very long but my love of yoga did. For many years I practised yoga on a mainly physical level, getting on the mat, cracking out some asana (physical postures) and enjoying a sleep at the end of class.

In my twenties, I very much enjoyed partying and clubbing with my friends. Yoga wasn't a priority for me, just something that I did. I began to teach yoga to friends and family for free and I started to really, really love yoga. I still partied, but yoga gradually crept up on me and became a fundamental part of who I am.

Everybody does yoga, every single day. Yoga has never been alien to us. It's a way of life. We have been doing it since we were babies. Whether it's the Cat Stretch to strengthen our spine and release our stiff backs or Wind-Relieving pose to 'boost digestion', if you look around you, you will always see people doing some physical form of yoga throughout the day.

Yoga means union, union of body and mind. This is why yoga is integral to the Birth ROCKS concept. I'd like to explain why the way that we think about and approach birth (our mind) affects how our resulting birth actually is (in our body.)

The other obvious union, is that of mother and child. Yoga is our natural state of being when we are pregnant. We are one with our unborn child. Sometimes it can take us a while for us to understand what that really means and this is part of our journey towards becoming a mother.

Yoga is always about looking inside yourself and finding out about the real you. By practising awareness and by understanding our true self, as we do when we practice yoga, we can prepare for birth with honesty and excitement. I keep saying it, but I really mean it!

I want you to use this book to begin your journey of self-discovery. To really get to grips with and to get to know YOU, before the most important event of your life. Yoga was for me was a pathway to self-discovery and I hope this book will be the first step towards yours.

So even if you never intend to step on a yoga mat, by reading this book and by starting to realize that life is no longer all about you any more, means that you are already practising yoga.

What can I expect from this book?

Hopefully, some common sense. This is not a pregnancy or birth 'bible' but a good honest overview of what to expect and some top tips on how to best prepare for your own unique birth. This book passes no judgement on any choices that you may make for your birth, but offers you support and a big virtual hug if you need one.

Why Birth ROCKS

Birth Rocks came about as a consequence of my first birth. I prepared for my birth using a well-known birth hypnosis programme (which I also used to teach to other mummies) and I was 100% prepared to be silent, peaceful and pain free during my birth. I practiced my 'techniques' religiously every day for nine months, and then my birth was nothing like I had planned.

Now I have to qualify this and say that I had the most amazing, beautiful, natural and speedy birth (about 5 hours from start to finish.) So what was the problem? Well, I didn't look like the serene ladies in the birth videos, that was for sure.

I made noise. I made a LOT of noise and I was loud and I writhed around. I even mooed like a cow for a large amount of my birthing time. I said random things to the midwives and my husband: "Mike you better make sure those bin bags are gone from the front door by the time I get home!"

My birth was at worst uncomfortable but mainly just damn hard work. At times I was meditative, breathing deeply, loudly, oblivious to anyone other than my baby, absorbed in my birth. Other times I was pumping with adrenaline talking to my baby: "Come on wee guy!! We can do this, come on wee man I love you, I love you so much!"

I had the natural birth I had hoped and planned for. Not every mother has that. So why did I still feel, to some extent, that I had 'failed?' I have years of training as a yoga teacher, with a daily meditation practice and I practised my 'birthing techniques' every evening without fail.

Why was I not silent like the mothers in the birth videos? Why was I so undignified making crazy noises and sitting on the toilet for 2 hours?? Why didn't my placenta detach from my womb at the end? What was wrong with me that all of these other women had peaceful, silent births and I couldn't shut up? My birth was amazing, the most tremendously spiritual experience of my life. But it wasn't like the picture.

Having taught birth hypnosis myself, I had subconsciously always thought that anyone who didn't achieve their picture perfect silent birth either:

- Didn't practice enough;
- Was weak;
- Had been subject to special circumstances.

Here I was, with no special circumstances, probably over practiced and didn't consider myself weak. I just couldn't keep quiet during birth!!

I began to think about the women I had taught over the years and around half of those mummies had silent, peaceful, drug free births. The rest of the mums had a range of outcomes.

Some women had special circumstances which had resulted in interventions and/or using pain medication. You can't plan everything for birth and sometimes special circumstances arise. Other mums had experienced pain during birth and had gone on to request drugs for pain relief. Some mums experienced pain but had continued on to have a drug free birth. A lot of these mums had practised their techniques on a daily basis. There was no physiological reason why some women should feel pain and not others. But it wasn't the birth in the picture. It wasn't the birth I had shown people in the videos or told them about.

After the birth, I would meet up with mums and speak to them about their birth and their experiences. Had it 'gone well?' (Were they silent, pain free and looking radiant afterwards?) Or had it 'not gone quite to plan?' (A noisy birth or a birth where drugs or interventions had been required?) I could hear women try to 'justify' or explain why they'd made noise or had used pain relief medication. I could hear the guilt in their voices, as if they had somehow wronged their baby or let them down by doing these things. I couldn't bare it!!

Here were women, mothers, with beautiful new babies who had gone through the most amazing experience of their lives, who were now suffering extreme birth guilt because their birth didn't match the pretty picture. And some women do have a silent, still, peaceful birth. But not everyone does!

So in writing Birth ROCKS and in creating this birth preparation programme, I have set out to put the record straight. I'd like to be clear from the start:

- All women are entitled to a beautiful birth: Silent or noisy!
- Birth guilt sucks: all births are equal, no matter what they looked like.
- All mothers and babies are unique and should be respected as such.
- Every birth is unique.
- Birth is not something to dread. We should be able to look forward to birth with love and excitement!
- Birth is not a competition. There are no prizes for 'the best birth.'
- Birth is hard work but rewarding.

Women, Birth & Mass Media Hysteria

Over the centuries, birth has become the most dreaded event in a women's life. In today's media, frequent images of pain, blood and screaming are being seen as the standard of childbirth today. Programmes such as *'One born every minute'* perpetuate this image of birth, traumatising women further by making it appear to be a real life insight into birth.

The majority of women have come to expect massive trauma while giving birth. This has pushed many birthing mothers towards taking advantage of the medical world's range of interventions now available. Choosing from a veritable buffet of drugs or opting to miss out on vaginal birth altogether and electing to have baby birthed through Caesarean section. It's no wonder that we are queuing up for an 'easy way out' of this horrific thing that is happening to us...

In recent years however, there has been a resurgence of women seeking to find out more about birthing naturally across the Western World. Women are attempting to reclaim their birth right: to birth without intervention, without drugs and often birthing out-with the hospital environment or even in water.

I'd like to be clear at this point that I am not pushing natural birth. I had a beautiful, natural birth myself but not everyone has or wants that as an option. This books is written without judgement and support for all women and all circumstances. However, pregnant women are seeing natural, alternative or holistic birthing options becoming more mainstream and widely available to them. Women are starting to realize that actually, natural birth could be the easiest, fastest and most rewarding option all round!

Different mediums allow women to educate themselves on the non-medical aspects of birthing through the internet, books, TV and film. More and more women are aware of the work of doulas (birth companions), many training formally to become birth companions and to help other women in this way. This inspiring push towards reclaiming birth is finally, allowing women to have real options and to make decisions about their birth, out with the generally accepted model of hospital birth.

Which birth is for me?

There are hundreds of birthing programmes and techniques that mothers can turn to, some promising more than others. Birth Hypnosis classes are one genre of childbirth preparation that has become very popular in recent years. Many of these programmes promise pain free and trance like births. Other programmes lead women to believe that achieving an orgasm during birth is a common and readily available option. Each new programme has a promise that their technique will make sure that mother has her perfect birth.

But isn't this just as dangerous as scaring women with stories of blood and gore? Are women being set up to fail?

Many birthing programmes deal with mothers who don't have the promised pain-free, silent birth by questioning them on what they 'hadn't done properly.' Had they practiced their hypnosis every single day? No? Then this is why their birth was not 'up to scratch.' No room for negotiation, the blame firmly being directed back to mother for not meeting their birthing standards.

Surely this is not a positive move towards empowering women. Making them believe that if they did not meet this new accepted standard of birth (silent, peaceful, orgasmic or pain free.) That it must in some way be their fault? That they had failed themselves and their child by causing this 'traumatic' birth?

I am in no way saying that birth hypnosis is not a valid technique for birthing mothers. Birth Hypnosis (as the inferred example) is an excellent option to offer for confidence, comfort and pain relief during birth. But it does not work for everyone and is not a 'cure all.' Of the many women that I taught birth hypnosis to over the years, fifty per cent had the beautiful blissful births that they hoped for and fifty per cent did not.

Why doesn't my birth look like that?

One birth hypnosis mother I worked with always sticks in my mind. She had practised her self-hypnosis techniques religiously, every day. The mother in question had a perfectly normal birth, a natural vaginal birth at home with no medical intervention or drugs and a beautiful healthy baby. When I spoke to her after the birth, she was devastated that she did not 'look like the women in the birth videos' and had made noise during the birth instead of remaining peaceful and silent. I do not believe this woman ever forgave herself, no matter how many times I reassured her that every birth is different. She would often say to me: 'Why couldn't I give birth like that? What did I do wrong?' It was at this point that I realized for certain, that I could not continue to offer one technique as the answer for ever person in every birth situation.

One size does NOT fit all

Every woman and every birth is unique and there is no fix-all option or cure for birthing. Drugs may not be the healthiest option for mother and baby, but neither is promising a mother a birth which may never become a reality for her and may cause her to harbour birth guilt. Birth is hard work and it may even hurt, but it is without a doubt, the most amazing and empowering experience that any woman is ever likely to have. Birth is worth every single minute of the effort. I am unable to describe the birth of my own son as painful, as I found it to be ecstatic. The sheer joy of meeting my little man face to face erased every memory of discomfort before it even existed.

It is my belief that birth preparation and education should be realistic. By this I do not mean presenting mothers with a list of interventions or drugs available. I don't think running through a list of catastrophic circumstances which may never arise is helpful either. Why put even more negative connotations into mothers mind? If mothers choose to educate themselves about birth, then their time needs to be spent positively. Clearly making false promises and setting standards of what is a good or bad birth is not positive or conducive to a happy birth experience either.

Birth preparation needs to have a strong focus on self-discovery. We cannot teach mothers how to give birth. Women already know how to give birth. What we can do, is to facilitate the journey of self-discovery with mothers and parents to be. To help them understand how they usually cope with new experiences and potentially stressful situations in everyday life. This knowledge can help parents translate these coping techniques into a birthing scenario. How do they normally react to discomfort or pain? What usually gives them comfort or relief?

I believe that we are in birth as we are in life and that what comforts us today, will comfort us during birth. This journey within, this getting to know and understand yourself, is essential in discovering how you can remain comfortable while birthing. We need to focus on opening up to the possibility of a joyful, comfortable and even ecstatic birth, without making mothers' false promises or assigning blame to those who don't meet the perfect birth criteria.

We cannot account for special circumstances arising during birth which necessitate medical intervention or mean that you may not have the birth that you hoped for. I believe that the role of birth preparation is not to give you a list of facts and figures, but to help you discover what you already know deep within yourself. Uncovering your real feminine strength (cheesy but true) that is integral to being a woman, that has been sullied by excessive intervention, propaganda and false promises.

Yes but I don't really like pregnancy...

And that's okay. Not everyone has a glowing shiny experience of pregnancy. I didn't.

Real life pregnancy can come as a bit of a shock, even if the pregnancy has been planned. I know that having wanted a baby for years and having worked with women who had beautiful pregnancies and births, I was quite taken aback by the often nauseating day to day realities of pregnancy.

I had envisioned myself floating around in white yoga clothing, cradling my growing bump, looking serene and bonding with my baby in utero, as I had often talked to other mothers about. I did not see myself with my head in a bucket every day and carrying a quickie sick bag everywhere for the majority of my pregnancy. This was the reality of the situation.

I suffered from hyperemesis gravidarium (or extreme pregnancy induced nausea and vomiting) from around six weeks gestation which lasted until I was almost eight months pregnant. So the floaty white outfits were a no-go straight away!

Why so sick?

The constant sickness was a real shocker for me. What happened to my perfect pregnancy and birth?? I knew how to take care of myself before conception and during pregnancy. I had mentored so many other mothers through peaceful pregnancies and beautiful births, so what had happened to my vision of pregnancy perfection? But like everything in life, pregnancy and birth are often not as we planned, even if we do 'know it all.'

NOT a pretty picture

The sickness really took its toll and the extensive yoga that I imagined I would practice every day, often consisted of me lying on my yoga mat having a hormonal sob at the injustice. With a bucket to hand, just in case. Being a yoga teacher and at the time, having a six day a week ashtanga practice, this was a major change for me. And not a pleasant one. I had always told mothers 'pregnancy is not an illness' and here I was, vomiting and unable to attend my place of work on a regular basis.

This was not working out to be the perfect, blissful pregnancy that I preached about oh-so-often. I started to doubt what I had been telling mums. Was it all a lie? Was pregnancy horrible? Was birth going to be even worse? Had the people who had taught me actually been crazy??

Find tips and tricks to make you feel better

As the weeks passed, the nausea didn't really get much better. But I continued my yoga practice, gently building up my strength again, practising slow, deep ujjayi breathing and easing slowly out of my downward dog.

I started to manage the nausea and vomiting a little better as the pregnancy progressed. I sported sea sickness acupuncture bands at all times (I think I had 10 pairs by the end of the pregnancy in a range of jaunty colours.) I only ever took them off to jump quickly into the shower and then quickly back on again. If I was longer than five minutes I would be sick, so I know that they worked for me.

Cheesy Wotsits were also my constant companion during the nauseous times. A very strange treatment, recommended to me by a local herbalist. I have never eaten them before and have never had the desire to eat them again unsurprisingly. The odd thing was that even the smell of the cheesy wotsits took away the sickly feeling, it really worked. An emergency packet of cheesy wotsits could keep the sickness at bay for at least an hour and so I would be buying multipacks at all hours of the day in my ever growing handbag.

As I started to find my own little tips and tricks, and as I was able to do a little more yoga, I started to feel more in control of my pregnancy and of what was happening to my body. I began to accept the fact that every day brought with it, a lot of vomiting. I started to see the funny side. I would be walking down the street with my friends chatting away and then have to 'excuse myself' to be sick in a bin, and then continue on my chat again. My friend said I was the sickest, happiest person she knew. I'm sure there is a compliment in there somewhere.

Enjoy your pregnancy, no matter what it looks like

I had preconceived idealistic ideas of what pregnancy was going to be like. It hadn't occurred to me that the 'glowing' women in my yoga classes were all having lovely, healthy, vomit free pregnancies. The ladies I didn't meet, were probably the poor sods being sick in a bucket at home like me. I suppose this gave me a very one sided view of pregnancy, the same way an anaesthetist and provider of epidurals would have a very one sided view of birth, seeing only the mothers who were experiencing a lot of pain.

My pregnancy wasn't the one that I dreamed of, but it was still my pregnancy and I was still going to have my own beautiful little baby to love and care for at the end of it.

Bond with your bump and slow down

I talked constantly to my bump (much to the amusement of work colleagues), singing songs and stroking my belly. I loved feeling my little man moving around, feeling him grow stronger and bigger. Meditation and travelling within to chat with my little man, became such an important aspect of my yoga practice during my pregnancy, as much of the time I couldn't manage any physical practice.

I learned to listen to my body. I accepted that my body no longer wanted to practice dynamic yoga every morning. I swapped my vigorous yoga sessions for a few gentle, aware postures which felt good for me and my baby. I gave into the early evening naps that my body so craved when I came home from work. I ate healthily (when the food would stay put) and changed to a liquid vitamin supplement with folic acid that my stomach could tolerate, instead of the horrible bulky tablets.

Remember that pregnancy ROCKS!

I learned that pregnancy is not always perfect, but neither is it a burden. My sickness was reassurance that my baby boy was taking hold and growing strong inside me.

Acceptance was the key for me, and this is what I try to teach to mothers who come to my classes during pregnancy. It could be nausea, it could be accepting that you can't run marathons anymore, or that you have to slow down and you don't really want to be in a blaring nightclub at 5 a.m. anymore. Every woman has an aspect of pregnancy or motherhood that wasn't what she expected. This doesn't make you a bad person; it's just new and takes some time to get used to.

Surrender to motherhood.

We need to allow ourselves to surrender to motherhood. Women today are expected to achieve all manner of feats while pregnant: keep working, go to aerobics, prepare dinner, and look after other kids… the list is endless.

The thing that makes us strong, the thing that makes us mothers, is our ability to sacrifice what we want in exchange for what's best for our child. The word surrender has a connotation of weakness. Surrendering to pregnancy doesn't mean you are weak; it means you are a strong and loving mother listening to what her body and baby need. Give yourself what you need during pregnancy, whether its sleep, some time off work, or cheesy wotsits. And please, please forgive yourself if you don't have that perfect, blissful pregnancy that we see on TV commercials.

Even though I wanted a baby so much, I didn't want to be sick every day. By reaching a place where I accepted that this was my story, my pregnancy and my way, I found absolute joy in my new prenatal yoga practice and in pregnancy. I went on to have an amazing birth and I will never forget the first moment I looked my little man in the eyes. So no matter how swollen your ankles or how creaky your pelvis becomes, I guarantee you that it's worth every minute.

Sophie's Pregnancy

Sophie is a first time mum from Belfast. She is pregnant with her first child and is six months in…

For as long as I can remember I have wanted to be a mum, and now that I am starting my seventh month of my pregnancy I am almost there! I have looked forward to being pregnant for a long time, and have over the years found myself indulging on reading articles, books and any other medium I can get my hands on to find out as much as I possibly can about pregnancy, birth and babies. As a YogaBellies teacher, I have spent so much time around pregnant women and new mums and now I am in the same position. I really feel that I have grown as a teacher and my personal experience has added to my knowledge and empathy.

Pregnancy for me has been a wonderful experience but I also feel that it has not been easy and makes me admire women who have had 3 or more babies! I have loved being able to experience so many new things that I have never experienced before, such as that first positive pregnancy test and telling my wonderful husband our amazing news. For the first few weeks, I felt that I was harbouring the most wonderful secret and I was getting so excited about being able to tell everyone. I kept looking at other pregnant women's bumps and almost wanting to let them know that I was part of their "club" too but I kept quiet in those early weeks.

The first few weeks were a time of quite considerable stress for me. I felt very vulnerable as I couldn't tell people before 12 weeks "just in case" something went wrong, and around 6 weeks, I unexpectedly starting to bleed heavily and I feared the worst. Thank goodness baby was strong and decided to stay with us and settle into its home for the next 8 months or so, but I really started to question this silence that has been placed upon us by society during the first trimester. I strongly feel that this is a time where women should be supported through the early days, and have people around them who are able to offer support, guidance and words of experience no matter the outcome of the pregnancy.

The pressure that was placed upon my husband and I, when we feared the worst was crushing. It made both of us realise that we loved our baby from the very start; as soon as we got that positive pregnancy test result. Of course our love has grown over time, but it really was there from the very beginning and when we saw our tiny little baby at our 12 week scan. It was such an amazing and life changing experience. I just remember being so overwhelmed that baby was back flipping and somersaulting around in there and I couldn't feel a thing!

As the weeks went by, I was noticing a beautiful roundness in my belly, and I was waiting with anticipation for those first kicks. I started to feel something around 15 weeks but wasn't too sure what it was as it felt like little bubbles popping in my tummy. Around a week later I was sure that it was our little baby testing out their legs. I remember my husband being upset that he couldn't feel the kicks when he placed his hand on my tummy at that stage, but he didn't have to wait long! I think it is so very hard for men to truly bond with their babies in that early stage, because all they see is their weary partner who has perhaps been vomiting continuously for the past number of months. They feel no kicks, their bodies aren't changing, all they see is their partner changing, and during the first trimester it is usually for the worst! Fortunately I didn't get one moment of morning sickness but was overwhelmed with tiredness, something that I really struggled to come to terms with.

I have always exercised and been fit and had a healthy appetite, and during my first trimester I felt as if I didn't know myself any more. I had no energy, my yoga mat lay on the floor almost neglected and all I wanted to do was sleep. I really felt that I was struggling through each day, simply going through the motions before I could get back to bed again and sleep once more, not the Sophie that anyone knew. I woke up one morning around 10 weeks pregnant and felt as if my world had come back to life again. My energy levels were up, my interest in food had returned and most importantly for me, I was able to get back to my yoga practice!

Something which I find difficult with being pregnant is that you are meant to get on with life as if nothing is different. You get up; you go to work and plough on with life. The difference is that everything is different! That is why I adore teaching pregnancy yoga because it is the one time in the week that mums get together to celebrate this incredible time and the journey that they are currently embarking upon. It is very hard to focus on the task at hand whenever your little one is tap dancing inside of you, bouncing on your bladder or swinging on your ribs in everyday life

I love being pregnant, and I can't wait to see this tiny little person in a few months' time. To feel someone growing inside you is a life changing experience. When baby is born and in my arms I know that I will still miss that feeling. I have loved nourishing my body with foods that are beneficial for both of us, and loved our daily yoga practise together helping to guide us towards our birth building and a sense of strength, stamina and also calmness and ease. I truly do not know how I could cope throughout pregnancy without yoga to guide me. It has been my absolute saviour as it always has. It has been so empowering to know that the yoga that I am practising at this time is for both of us, and that with each breath I take I am breathing for my baby too. Yoga has kept me calm and contented, and made me so aware that my baby is a part of me and that I need to be calm for the both of us.

I have enjoyed so much preparing myself for the birth, something that I started to do as soon as I found out that I was pregnant. It baffles me that women plan their weddings to the nth degree to ensure that the "most important day of their lives" goes off without a hitch, but they don't prepare to the same extent for the arrival of their babies. Yes women may attend antenatal classes and listen to what midwives have to say but many are much more excited about their new prams or their babies beautiful little clothes. Of course this plays a considerable part, but so much focus is placed upon when the baby is here, and not the birth, the most important aspect of how the baby actually gets here. People prepare for weddings and train for marathons and birth should be treated in the exact same way.

My preparation for the birth has consisted of reinforcing my excitement of the occasion of my physical birth. I can safely say that I have no fear whatsoever about bringing our baby into the world, I just can't wait to experience childbirth as I feel that it is a moment to be celebrated and looked forward too as opposed to dreaded and feared. Throughout my pregnancy I have never ceased to be amazed at how my body knows exactly what it is doing as it grows our baby and prepares my body for its arrival. The female body is truly miraculous, and women are so strong and powerful to be able to achieve this. I feel a sense of completeness now, almost as if I am allowing my body to fulfil the purpose for which it has been created.

Despite the fact that I have loved my pregnancy, I have also struggled with acute back pain from an old injury which pregnancy hormones have brought out. This has made it difficult at times and I have had to work very hard to not let my physical back pain mentally get the better of me, but once again the yoga has helped me to focus my mind and honour myself in the moment. I have always been the sort of person who ploughs ahead and perhaps my back pain is a way of showing me that I need to slow down and savour the moment, because a pregnancy is so short and I will never experience this pregnancy again. Pregnancy is a gift that keeps on giving, and I can't wait for the gift of our baby to come gently into this world and into our arms.

Does it hurt? And why Fear creates Pain

"I would say the most surprising thing that I learned throughout my labour, was my newfound ability to manage pain, having previously been known to be a bit of a drama Queen with the slightest bump, trip or stubbed toe. I had this feeling of power and strength and focus, to let my body go with it, and to breathe, just breathe.........breathe"
Andreina O'Neill

Honestly, does it hurt??

Everyone experiences birth differently but I can put my hand on my heart and say that I cannot describe my birth as painful. It was hard work, lots of hard work and I think the comparison to running a marathon is a very good one. Hard work and rewarding.

This is not the prettiest description of what childbirth feels like, but for me this is the most accurate description. It's like having a big poo. Have you ever been constipated and been about to pass a big poo and thought: "Actually this is going to nip. I'm not sure if I can do this. Oh no, this poo is going to be sore!"

And just when you think it's so unbearable that you cannot possibly pass the poo, the poo comes and it's all over. And you think to yourself, "That wasn't so bad after all."

Childbirth, for me, was like that. It's the perception of pain and the anticipation of pain that makes something painful. Just as we talked about earlier, the Fear (of the big poo/of giving birth), creates Tension in the body (holding in the poo/holding in baby) that makes it Painful (painful poo passing/painful childbirth.)

Everyone has different experiences and perceptions of pain during childbirth. This is nothing to do with your 'pain threshold' or how 'strong' a person you are. No-one can judge anyone else's experience of birth. Only you are in your birth and only you know how you feel. So if you honestly feel the best way for you to cope with the sensations of childbirth is to take drugs, then take drugs. But please, please keep an open mind at the onset and give natural birth a try. You may find it works out pretty well for you ☺

The Fear Tension Pain Cycle

"It didn't hurt. It wasn't meant to, was it, doctor?"

When Dr. Grantly Dick-Read attended the birth of a poor English girl in the 1900's, this is what she said to him when he offered her chloroform for pain relief. When he asked her why she did not want the drugs, this was her reply.

Dr. Grantly Dick-Read was taken aback when he went on to witness the woman give birth without discomfort or pain medication. This birth set him on the path to looking at childbirth in a whole new way, as a normal physiological process instead of the terrifying painful experience it had been come to be seen as. When his book, "Childbirth without Fear" was published in the1930's, the book was disregarded as nonsense, but is now seen as a vital turning point in attitudes towards natural birth and childbirth as a normal, natural process and not an illness. This is a really fantastic book about childbirth which I would highly recommend.

Dr Dick-Read continued to study birthing women and attempted to find out what made one birth experience so different from another. He came to the conclusion that the more a woman feared childbirth, the tenser she would become and as a result of this, she would have a more painful childbirth.

When we become scared, our bodies go into 'fight or flight' mode. This means that the body releases a hormone called adrenaline which helps us to act fast and move away from dangerous situations. It diverts all of the blood and oxygen in the body away from 'non-vital' areas such as the uterus, to 'vital areas' such as the brain, arms and legs to give you more strength and speed to escape danger. The adrenaline which is produced can slow down or stop labour all together. This fight or flight mode has obvious benefits in the wild. So if you think about a labouring zebra (random) giving birth in the wild and a lion approaches, the zebra will go into 'fight or flight' mode and their body will literally halt birthing, often pulling the baby zebra back up into the womb, allowing the zebra to become mobile and get away from the attacking lion. Your chances of being attacked by a Lion during childbirth are (hopefully!) very small.

However, our bodies still work in exactly the same way. If we are scared of birth, our body will produce adrenaline. During birth our body naturally tries to expel baby, but the adrenaline produced slows down and stalls birthing. Therefore we have two systems fighting each other. We cannot 'relax and let go' and be stressed at the same time. Fact.

What physically happens when I'm scared of giving birth?

Okay now for the science bit. The uterus is made from two layers (well three but we only need to know about two) of muscles that go in two different directions. One layer runs from the top to the bottom and the other goes around the sides. During labour, the "first" set of muscles contract to push the baby down and pull the cervix back. After your baby is born, the other set of muscles contract to pull the cervix and uterus back into place.

If you become scared of giving birth, the muscles around the sides of your uterus contract and tighten. This means that your uterus is working against itself - one set of muscles is trying to open the cervix while the other set of muscles is trying to close the cervix. This can make for a very long, painful, and unproductive labour. I'm sure you've heard of 'failure to dilate.' That's exactly what this is.

This came to be known as the "Fear-Tension-Pain" cycle is because it works in a cycle: fear of birthing, makes the body tense which makes birthing painful.

Preparing to Relax during Birth

Relaxation holds the key to managing pain in labour, but you must try to understand what works for you during everyday life. Remember what worked wonders for your friend, may not work for you. That's why it's important to know what soothes and calms you now and work from there. Your Birth ROCKS Mentor can help you understand what your natural coping style is which will be a good indication of what will work for you during childbirth.

Make sure you take time out to learn and master techniques to relax your body, and to keep you calm during the waves. Remember that relaxing actually takes practice. Even if you have tried relaxation methods such as yoga or meditation in the past, chances are your first response to pain (back ache, leg cramps, standing on a plastic dinosaur) is to tense that part of your body.

If you have Braxton Hicks (practice) contractions this is a great time to get practising. Practice in various situations, try out different birthing positions and see if you can relax through the pain.

Build it up. Start to increase the amount of time you spend relaxing every day until you able to relax for at least half an hour. If you even have five or ten minutes to practice, this will all be of benefit.

During the birth, your waves will at most, last up to around 90 seconds. You will probably find that you want to relax and get back into 'the zone' between the waves.

So how do I get rid of my fear of giving birth?

This is what we want to focus on. Now we have explained the effect of fear on childbirth, clearly we want to now identify and resolve any fears you may have of birthing or becoming a parent. These are the kind of issues that if left unresolved, could pop up during childbirth.

This is why we say that pregnancy and birth are a journey of self-discovery. It's time to be completely honest with yourself and your birth partner about who you are, what are you are scared of and what you need to move past this and to be able to enjoy birth.

Being honest with yourself and your birth partner

Getting to know and understand you is the most important part of honest birth preparation. Both you and your birth partner should be honest with each other too. Your choice of birth partner is very important and will have a huge impact on your comfort and ability to relax during childbirth. For example, if your birth partner is also your life partner or husband or wife, then have you asked them about how they feel about being at the birth or if they in fact even want to be at the birth? I hear you gasp in horror.

"If I'm going to have to be at the birth, then they sure as hell are!"

I hear mums to be say when I dare to suggest this. But think about this again. If dad (let's say dad for argument's sake but you know that I am referring to any life partner) is terrified by the prospect of being at the birth, is this really going to be productive, useful or comforting for you or them?

Men and Childbirth

Having men at the birth is a very new concept and many people don't think it's a great idea. As recently as the 1970's, men were not allowed to come into the birthing environment and it was an 'all women' area. Personally, I don't think that's a bad thing and I'll give you a personal example from the birth of my son.

My husband is a medic and has been present at childbirth before and operates on people on a daily basis, so it did not even occur to me that being at the birth would be an issue. I'm pretty sure I didn't ask him.

The first time that I realized that Mike had completely freaked out, was when we were getting into the car to go to the hospital. He said, "It's all going to be fine the hospital is only ten minutes away." I think he said this about twenty times.

During the birth, my poor husband had a look of shock and fear on his face the whole way through. The midwives and I asked him if he'd like a seat or maybe a glass of water. Mike was in shock. This is not to say that he was not amazingly supportive and lovely, as he always is, but the scared expression on his face (on the face of a man who is at all times completely composed and in control of the situation), said to me that there was something wrong that he wasn't telling me. This made me worry. This created tension in my body and I had to keep asking him, "Is there something I don't know? Is everything okay?"

I had an amazing peaceful, euphoric (often very noisy) birth and that I could not have hoped for a better experience. When we discussed it later, Mike said that he felt as if he was in a medical situation that he had no control over. My strange mooing noises and writhing, which are completely normal during birth, made him feel that he should be doing something, when really all I was doing was relaxing into birth in my own unique way. Being a medic, my husband viewed the situation as medical and as there were no medical interventions, it all seemed alien to him.

I don't think I would want to put him through that again, and I don't think it would be helpful for me to be worrying about how he felt during the birth again. You may be thinking, I still definitely want my partner to be there and that is absolutely fine, but I do ask that you have a think and an honest and frank discussion about it beforehand. My husband is the best husband and dad in the world (yes I'm a bit biased) but I think next time, it's going to be all girls present at the birth. There is something reassuring about an all-woman environment, women helping women.

Gemma Cassidy Broderick's First Birth

Nikki is a nurse living in Glasgow who attended Birth ROCKS sessions. Nikki had a high BMI and was indicated as 'high risk' during pregnancy yet went on to have a beautiful natural birth with her first baby at 42 weeks using, only gas and air.

I went to Nicolas class with an open mind. My husband was not so keen on the "Hippy mumbo jumbo," but if it works then great. I thoroughly enjoyed my class and Nicola (Birth ROCKS Mentor) is a credit to the company and the women she teaches.

I went into labour at 40+2. I had been using my birthing ball to bounce and rock, lots of walking; eating pineapple, drinking raspberry leaf tea and I fell in love with clary sage and would sit and sniff that at night.

By Monday the 25th of February I was a week 'overdue.' I was seriously fed up. I was bored and lonely with Kevin being at work. I had "No twinges" or so I thought and my Induction was now booked in for the 28th. My mum was coming down from my home town 12 miles away the week prior (to my due date) but had been sick and so had stayed away. I kept asking her, "When are you coming?" over the weekend and she kept replying whenever you need me. Finally on Sunday, I said to her, "Please just come tomorrow, I'm bored and need someone to come out with me"

My mum arrived at lunchtime and I wanted to go and have my nails done and she was more than happy to do this and suggested we do it on Tuesday. However, I wanted them done right there and then and so 45 minutes later and we were in the salon. We had a quick bite to eat after the manicure and then a trip to Asda for some supplies. Now normally at this time of day at around 4 or 5 pm I start to feel an ache in my lower back, like a postural pain, as if I have been leaning over in the wrong way all day. I never thought it was any more than just my normal pregnancy aches.

We headed home and had dinner and I just couldn't settle. I felt a bit restless, and didn't quite know what to do with myself, so at 10pm that evening we all went to bed. I don't think I slept too deeply and at 11pm I remember getting a period-like pain which came and went. Then a couple minutes later I had another and then another, then another. I still didn't really think much of it at this point but it woke me from my sleep. Shortly afterwards, I felt the urge for the toilet (a number 2!) By this point I was on the toilet and the pains suddenly increased in severity and there was a bright red clotted bloody show. Now I knew this was it for sure.

I phoned maternity assessment to let them know and by this point the pains were coming very close together and my breathing is very audible to the midwife on the phone. She asks me to come in for assessment. I am happy to do this so off we go.

On route in the car, while I am sitting down the sensations are very intense. Sitting down is hell and I don't like it at all. Thankfully we arrive 10 minutes later and then I'm on the bed being examined by a lovely midwife that I get to know a little better over the next 36 hours. It transpires that my cervix is high, posterior and not dilated. With the reassurance of the midwife, I flick into positive mental attitude mode and try to take best out of the situation. My cervix is not as dilated as I had hoped, but at least things have started. Each contraction is one step closer. I had prepared myself for a 2 day labour and we go home until things start to move along.

At home I find very quickly that I don't like to sit. I need to stand or walk through each contraction (I don't mind calling them contractions/pains or anything medical as I'm a nurse and don't associate negativity with these words or the hospital.) The best position I can find is leaning over my breakfast bar, knees bent, and gyrating my hips in a figure of eight. Whilst I do this I am breathing in long and slow and then out for double (the full YogaBellies breath.) A breath taught by Nicola and which I use throughout my labour.

If I am sitting at the onset of a contraction I find I need to get up quickly to catch it, otherwise I can't get up and need to sit for the duration and its hell to sit through. At this point, I flash back to the class and the exercise where Nicola has us draw our birth. My picture showed me kneeling upright against the back of the bed. I'm starting to think that will be the case as sitting/lying down is not working for me.

This continues until 7am. The pains increased in severity and in frequency and so I phoned back in to speak to the midwife. At the back of my mind I'm just worried about getting stuck in rush hour traffic if I leave it any longer to go. I feared this would be the case and I knew that if I need to sit for any length of time in the car then I wouldn't be in control, so off we went again.

On arrival I am examined and am showing the same presentation. Argh! Okay so I take a step back and bring in the PMA again. I turn it around, things are still happening, I am still in labour and we are now X amount of contractions closer to meeting our wee one. The midwife gives me the option of staying in or going home. We decide to go home.

At this point I accept a painkiller and manage to snooze for 3 hours at home. Coincidently my contractions tail off.

Tuesday was spent bouncing on my ball, and walking through the pains the same as through the night. My hubby, mum and dad are all in the house, and we munch down a KFC for lunch not that I ate much of it. Later on that night, things slowly increase again and we decide to go out for a walk about 8pm in the pitch black and freezing cold. But the cold air is just perfect for me. Contracting often, I just walk it out and stop when needed and breathe them away. Easy peasy!

We get home and I remember thinking I wanted to have a bath and to wash my hair before I go back in, so now would be the time to do that. I manage to dry my hair and then the contractions are on the up. Now I have found that breathing in long low dulcet tones feels great. I find myself saying vowels... as in...
eeeeeeeeeeeeee...aaaaaaaaaaaaaaa.....ooooooo etc... and then sometimes I would say a word, and then think of all

the words that rhyme with that word. I.e. Joe, sow mow, low, and so on.

This came from nowhere, I hadn't planned it but it just came and it worked for me. One of the funny things is that after every single contraction I would yawn. Kevin never needed to ask if it was over, he just waited for my rhyming to stop and for me to yawn, then we would both have a good giggle and comment how you can be in so much pain one minute and not the next. This kept me going. My focus was that the contractions come and go. The will get worse then they go. Keep this in mind and it will be fine. I asked Kevin to remind me this when I was losing focus, "Tell me the pain will go" that's all I wanted to hear from him when things got tough.

By 2am, we are back in maternity assessment. On examination, I am now 3-4 cm dilated and I am delighted. The same lovely midwife then got me to sit on a backwards chair with lots of pillows and handed me the gas and air, which I loved! Gas and air rocks!

I felt it kept the pains at a great level as they were actually increasing in intensity. By 6:30 I was accepted by labour suite and we walked round. It felt like 2 minutes to me but Kevin reckons it took me around 15 minutes to get there.

When we got to the room, I stated straight away that I wanted to be upright and on my feet, but after having to be examined and having a contraction on the bed I found it very comfortable and so decided to just stay there. By this point I was 6 cm and was just delighted.

The midwife asks if I had an anaesthetic review and what the outcome had been: an epidural due to my BMI. The good news was that I did not want one nor did I need one. I was coping fine with the pain. I wasn't too tired and just simply did not want a catheter in so no epidural for me. Just as we were discussing this, the consultant and her team came in, and were surprised to see my smiling face and commented as such. She also reiterated that I was doing amazingly well and certainly did not need an epidural and walked back out within a couple of minutes. That gave me such a positive boost!

Over the next 20 min or so the contractions actually became really painful and this is where most of the course and my birth preparation kicked. My breathing continued to be deep and long, but now I was using my left hand to help me through. I will describe this as best as I can.

I had my finger and index finger together and imagined a needle and thread and with each contraction I did some sewing. I visualised pulling the thread up through my body and then out the other side. I also visualised Nicola as she was teaching this breath and her hand was the same way as mine now and all I could see was her, and the session where we did the breathing and visualisation. I then floated back to when she did the rainbow relaxation piece and floated myself, just remembering how relaxing it was listening to her.

I then noticed my breathing was becoming louder, like a grunting but through the mouth piece of my gas and air, which for some reason took me back into my dad's place of work. He was a butcher and used to freeze meat then cut it into cubes with a big saw and with every breath I took, the vibration of the mouthpiece and my tones reminded me of my days helping him out and having to listen to that damn saw. Very bizarre, but that's what happened.

At this point my midwives asked me if I practised yoga as they noticed my left hand and my good breathing practice and I started to tell them about Birth ROCKS, but was interrupted by a contraction!

Next came the pushing and this I hadn't prepared for! I found it very tough and difficult but go through but it was all over in 25 minutes and my wee darling arrived healthy, very bright and alert and I think she had a second or two of a gurgle, but didn't really cry. A very chilled out baby.

My fears at the start were that I would have to have epidural, only because I was "high risk" as I had a high BMI. I had a healthy pregnancy and attended every appointment as requested and did all test and scans and after the Birth ROCKS course, I kept a positive mind that my body would know what to do. I used my Oxytocin to relax and allow things to "open" and to allow baby to come, rather than stress and worry and tense up which in my mind, which shuts down the body and stops baby coming.

The main things that got me through were deep long breathing, visualisation, positive mental attitude and keeping mobile. I trusted that Nicola knew that I could do it, if that makes sense?

Most importantly, I really did love being in labour! The only thing is, for next time, I will prepare for the pushing as I found that challenging, but not enough to put me off doing it again.

Face the Fear and Do it Anyway

You don't have too many options here ladies. You are pregnant and you are going to give birth. So let's look at the options moving towards birth.

Option 1: Pretend it isn't happening.

Ignore the fact you are pregnant, carry on as normal and turn up on the day and put your birth in the hands of the hospital staff. Prepare to be offered all of the drugs and to have lots of intervention resulting in a C-section.

Option 2: Take the drugs.

Read as many books as possible about everything imaginable that could go wrong. Make sure you hear every horror story there is about childbirth so that you have all the information and watch One Born Every Minute religiously, taking great care not to hide your eyes during the really gruesome bits. The more bad things you know about birth, the more you will be prepared right? Um....

Option 3: Plan for 'The Perfect Birth'

Sign up for a birth preparation course which promises you the perfect birth, orgasms during transition and absolutely pain free labour. Prepare to sneeze your baby out. Get ready to be a glowing, white dress wearing Earth Mother who breezes through birth and parenthood.

Option 4: Be Realistic but Optimistic

Respect that fact that you are pregnant. Carry on with as many normal activities as you are comfortable with, rest and relax when you need to, bond with your baby and allow yourself to enjoy pregnancy, vomit and all. Prepare for birth with honesty and excitement. Don't listen to horror stories, don't look at pictures of forceps and don't plan for tragedy.

Think about what comforts you now in every-day life. Get to know yourself and your birth partner and be honest with yourself. Make a plan for birth and be prepared for it to change on the day.

Be prepared for childbirth to be bloody hard work but also an amazing once (or twice, thrice...) in a lifetime experience that will blow your mind – in a good way! Feel lucky that you are getting to experience childbirth! Get excited and know that the majority of the time, childbirth can be without medical intervention. It may be peaceful, it may be messy or noisy, it may be all of these things, but it will definitely be entirely unique to you.

Listen to happy baby stories, always be positive and learn and read about the natural physiological aspects of childbirth. How birth feels; how to manage the sensations and how to be comfortable. Find out information that is actually going to be useful and understand that you are IN your birth, not at it.

You can probably realize that I am not suggesting you go for any of the first three options. Option four is what we are aiming for. Realistic, honest and very, very positive about giving birth.

What does tension feel like?

Let's look first of all at recognising tension in your body. Think about the different things that you do when you are tense:

- Do you hunch your shoulders and neck?

- Do you sweat? Shake? Turn red?

- Do you stammer? Become mute?

What tension feels like for you?

You need to be able to recognize tension in your body. It's very possible you are carrying a lot of tension right now, only you are so used to feeling it that you don't even recognize it anymore! Understanding and being able to recognize the difference between a tensed and a relaxed muscle is the best way to begin relaxation.

Try lying still on the floor or a chair and tensing and relaxing the different muscles in the body. This will give you a good idea of where you carry tension, and identify areas that need more help relaxing.

What makes you tense and how do you cope?

Think about times in the past when you have encountered a new or stressful situation. Maybe going to the dentist is something you really hate to do.

- How did the prospect of this make you feel? Consider the signs of physical tension in your body.
- How did you cope with this tension?

- What made it lessen or go away?
- What helps to relax you?

Your Birth ROCKS Mentor can help you identify the signs of tension in your body and also to recognize how you most effectively relieve that tension also try these exercises at home with your partner to get you started.

Identifying and Uncovering your Fears

"I was surprised at how me (and my body) at time just knew what to do to help me through! Along with gas and air!! And now I have an amazing baby boy ... Who's not so much of a baby anymore as that was nearly 20 months ago!"

Emma Lindsay Fitzsimmons

The Birth ROCKS process of releasing your fears involves first and foremost being honest with yourself and your partner and examining what you are scared of. Discuss this with your partner at length. Once we have identified our fears, then we can face them. We are then able to identify how tension presents itself in your body. We can begin to consider ways in which we can lessen or minimize these signs of tension.

We can then move on to looking those fears in the eye, being completely honest about what they are and how we can deal with them. Your Birth ROCKS Mentor can help you use different techniques to get these fears out in the open, but you can begin by considering the following:

Tackling your fears 'Head On'

Don't run away from or try not to think about the things that scare you about giving birth. I am not telling you to 'dwell on' things that may never happen which is just as counterproductive and I am not asking you to over analyse, but I am saying, let's be honest (there it is again) about your fears. Let's not shy away from them, let's take them on, challenge them and see what we can do to resolve them.

- What are you really scared of?

- Why are you scared of this?

- Is there any reason why this should happen?

- What is the worst that could happen?

- What can you do to make yourself feel better about this?

- Whatever you need to do, do it! Make a plan to make this fear go away so that you can move onwards and upwards!

For example, if you are terrified of having a C-section, why are you so scared of this particular procedure? Is there any medical indication at this stage why this should happen? Let's say there was a high chance of this due to medical reasons, what would this mean for you in terms of how would this differ from a 'normal' birth and how would your recovery change?

- What can you do to still make this the happy, peaceful birth you hoped for?

- What would make this situation better and more manageable for you and your baby and your partner?
  - What can you do to minimize the chances of this having to happen at all?

Michelle's First Birth: Baby Ethan Ashton James Anderson

Michelle's first baby Ethan was born back to back with signs of meconium but went on to have a natural birth.

Friday 7th October 2012, my mother's 52nd birthday, I woke up with a strong urge to go to the loo. (Number Two!) This happened to me a couple of times that morning. I thought to myself I must have upset my tummy from the Indian food I had eaten the evening before. Unknown to me, it was my body preparing itself for labour.

I decided to go for a shower around 10.00am to freshen up. 10.20am not long after getting out my shower, I felt, what I would describe as, a very strong tightening across my lower abdomen. This feeling lasted for around one minute and then to my relief, stopped. Wondering what just happened, I decided to go and tell my partner Allan all about it. However, shortly afterwards again, I felt another shooting sensation. "Allan" I said," I think this could be the start of my contractions...." and it was!

My contractions were lasting around 50 seconds to 1 minute every occurrence, and between 3-4 minutes apart. (We were using my phone to time them) I remember thinking how wonderful it felt in between contractions. I was amazed at how, one minute I was on the floor on all fours (hands and knees) rocking back and forth, and the next laughing with Allan about what was happening to us that morning. In between one of my contractions, I called my mum to wish her a happy birthday. Needless to say how ecstatic she was on the phone, when I told her I thought my baby was about to make an appearance on her birthday.

I was very mindful that the midwives at our antenatal classes had advised us to stay at home for as long as possible before heading to the hospital. I also remembered they had said 'or at least until your contractions were between 3-4 minutes apart' this worried me slightly as my contractions were coming every 3-4 minutes so early on. I decided to call the maternity assessment unit and let them know my contractions had started. They confirmed all sounded ok, and as already aware, to stay at home for as long as I can manage. At this stage I was comfortable and happy to stay at home.

Around 1pm I decided to walk to the kitchen to get myself a glass of water. Suddenly, out from nowhere ....Whoosh... my waters had broken all over the kitchen tiles. My friends laugh at me when I tell this story, as I always remember to tell them how pleased I was to make the decision to go downstairs at this time, as, if my waters had broken upstairs, it would have been a very difficult job for Allan to clean off the CREAM carpets!

I then called the maternity assessment unit again to update them on my progress. They believed as it had only been three hours from the start of my contractions, and the fact that I was able to speak to them through a contraction, that I was still at very early stages and advised that I could be sent back home again after my check-up. The check-up was to take place to confirm whether my waters had broken. At this stage I had a lot of pressure on my pelvis and it was difficult to remain upright on my two feet. The most comfortable position for me during my contractions was down on all fours, rocking back and forth. I was very worried at the thought of going to the hospital and having to be sent back home as I could barely walk with the pressure.

It took us around 20 minutes to get to the hospital. My mum met us there. My mum and Allan were going to be my birthing partners. I remember waiting around, for what felt like ages, in the maternity assessment, waiting to be examined. Eventually, when it was my turn, I remember dreading the thought of an examination. Especially, as it involved a speculum. During the examination I had another contraction. Soon the examination was over and the midwife told me I was 4 centimetres dilated. To my relief I knew that meant I didn't have to go home if I didn't feel up to it. However they then told me that there was some meconium in my waters and that I would have to be continuously monitored in the labour suite from then on, to allow them to keep an eye on the baby. This meant I couldn't have the water hospital birth I had hoped for. I was told that I had to prepare myself in the event that I had to be taken to theatre. I soon got a needle in my arm to prepare for a theatre delivery and was taken to the labour ward. At this stage I started to feel a little anxious about the 'what ifs'. However my mum and Allan soon helped me stop focusing on the negatives and to continue focusing on my breathing techniques and to try and relax as much as possible, just as I had learned through my I-hypo-birthing tools, my pre-natal yoga class (YogaBellies) and what I had read in Ina May Gaskin's book about childbirth.

To my surprise I was taken to a pleasant hospital room and allocated a midwife at the labour ward. I wasn't aware that a midwife was to be present at all times during my labour. (From watching One Born Every Minute during pregnancy, it was my understanding that the midwife just popped in now and then)

I was soon hooked up to a monitor to allow the midwife to keep an eye on baby. By this point I was getting very strong back pain. During an examination I was told baby was back to back. I didn't understand why the midwife was focusing on this or what complications this could bring. I did ask the midwife however she told me not to worry about it for now. Throughout my labour the only position I felt comfortable in was on all fours on top of the hospital bed. I remembered trying to stand a few times but my feet couldn't take the pressure and so I was on my knees most of the day. I was also unaware that throughout your labour – blood 'show' would be coming away from me – again why hadn't I seen this in OBEM? I thought this only happened at the pushing stage.

I started taking the gas and air to help ease the pressure. The next four hours (although time seemed to go past very quickly for me) was spent rocking on my knees, drinking water, having hot packs on my back, laughing with my mum and Allan, which all helped to ease the discomfort. During this time I was given another examination and told the baby was still back to back. Eventually, after repeatedly asking, the midwife explained that if the baby wasn't to turn on their own then I may need some assistance. I remember thinking to myself that will not be happening if I have anything to do with it!

10pm arrived and my final examination, to my relief I was told I was now fully dilated and the baby had managed to turn into the optimal position. My midwife explained she was going to leave me for another hour before asking me to push. At this point she took a break and another midwife entered the room. I remember having a good laugh and joke with this midwife. Soon my original midwife came back into the room and before I knew it, it was 10.50pm

At 10.55pm I got a very strong urge to push. This stage of labour was very different. At this stage I was so excited at the thought of meeting my baby. I remember also feeling slightly anxious at this stage, as I wasn't sure what to do or how I going to push this baby out. I had learned some breathing techniques through my pre-natal yoga class, which was meant to help reduce the chance of tearing and stiches. I remember listening to the midwife when she was explaining how to push. (Down onto your bum, holding your breath and pushing as hard as possible) however as much as I was pretending to listen to her, I focused on what I had learned in my yoga class known as 'breath out your baby'. The midwife kept asking me to stop breathing out and asking me to try and hold my breath; however this breath felt more natural to me. During crowning, I felt my baby's head on several occasions. Twenty minutes later, at 23.16 a beautiful baby boy, weighing 7lbs 2oz arrived naturally into this world, without a complication, tool or tear. All discomfort, burning sensations, contractions gone instantly. Wow!

My baby boy was immediately placed onto my chest. Skin to skin contact immediately as per my 'birth wish plan' my mum had called out and told me it was a boy when he made an appearance. I believe he lay there for around 15 mins before the midwife let Allan cut the cord. He didn't cry once, he just stared at me with his big eyes for which seemed like hours.

I have heard of having an orgasmic birth, I cannot say I had an orgasm during birth, but what I would say is, that when my baby arrived in my arms it felt as good as, even better than an orgasm !!!

The midwife typed up her notes in the background after delivering the placenta and checking for tears. My mum and Allan were on the phone, and I was enjoying my first moments with my beautiful baby boy. Ethan had a large egg shape lump on the back of his head – this was due to the amount of turning he had to do during labour. I had asked the midwife about feeding my baby, she helped try and get Ethan onto the breast but he wasn't ready. He wasn't rooting or looking for it, so in the end she told me it would be ok and that feeding doesn't always take place instantly.

I was so delighted to hear Ethan was a boy, not that I would have been disappointed if he was a girl, but I just had a feeling I was having a boy, and kept having mind images of me holding a baby boy.

Before leaving the room to go help with a delivery next door, the midwife took Ethan from me to check him over and weigh him. Before I knew it he was back in my arms. After having tea and toast, I went for a quick bath to freshen up and daddy and nana enjoyed some cuddles.

It was 3 am before I got into the post natal ward. Allan and my mum left me to get some rest. I could not sleep. All I wanted to do was stare at my baby boy. I was so conscious that I hadn't fed him yet. By this point he had fallen asleep. I called on a midwife and asked her about breastfeeding my baby, she told me not to worry too much as he was asleep and to call her when he had woken and that I should try and get some rest. As if! I couldn't go to sleep and leave this tiny little baby in his crib all by himself. Even though he was right beside my bed he felt a long distance away. I wasn't allowed to go to sleep with him in the hospital bed.

So in the end I got up and sat naked (top talk) with my dressing gown around us both and gave him lots of cuddles.

Before I knew it we were called for breakfast, Ethan was still sleeping by this point. After breakie, Ethan was given a wash and daddy came to see us. Ethan was covered in meconium and I hadn't realised. It was all in his hair, nails etc. The nurse had to change the water twice as he was so dirty. By this point he had of course woken up. A midwife came to help me with breastfeeding, whilst I awaited the arrival of my aunty Margaret (breastfeeding support worker)

Breastfeeding was more challenging than I had imagined, was told or had read about. Ethan would latch on and then within seconds would come off. When he managed to get something he would then get so frustrated and start screaming when he came off, that it was difficult to get him back on again. I remember thinking, this baby – who wasn't even a day old as yet, was a lot stronger than I expected him to be. He was pushing me away and I was frightened of hurting him in any way. He was getting something – that was the important thing. Lots of skin to skin contact and cuddles were also very important for us. As the day got on and the more we tried bf, the more upset I became. My aunt had arrived and was trying to reassure me that everything would be ok. Unfortunately when she was visiting, Ethan slept most of the time. She reminded me how small his tummy was and that what I was able to give him was more than enough. He was also full of mucus and so she explained that was properly making him feel full.

As the day got on I had to drip feeding colostrum into my baby's mouth, drop by drop. We kept trying to get Ethan to latch on properly, but after a few seconds he kept coming back off again which made him very upset. I was told by one of the nurses/midwifes that I had flat nipples. I didn't know the difference, to me they were normal looking nipples and so didn't realise different nipples caused challenges. I was told as they were so flat (soft) when baby was trying to latch on and that he wasn't able to get a proper grip.

I remained in hospital until the Thursday (had baby Sunday evening) Due to my breastfeeding challenges, I was told I

wasn't to get home until bf was going better. With a
mixture of short breast feeds and hand expressing, I was
managing to give my baby something, albeit to me seemed
like very little volumes. I was getting lots of encouragement
and support via telephone from my aunt. By day 3 I was
very emotional, the constant hand expressing and not being
able to feed my baby properly, was getting me down. That
evening, to my relief I was introduced to a new midwife
who told me I was going to stop expressing and that she
was going to help get this baby to express himself. She
spent a lot of time with us talking and guiding me, making
sure Ethan was positioned correctly. My positioning was
fine I was told it was just a matter on helping him stay on
that was the challenge. The next day I got the ok from the
doctors and was able to go home at last!

By the time I got home on the Thursday my boobs were
solid and full. Because of this, Ethan again then found it
hard to get a good grip of my breast/nipples (they basically
didn't want to move shape at all) I wasn't able to feed
Ethan successfully at all Thursday evening or Friday
morning. He started to develop what looked like jaundice;
he was becoming very sleepy. He hadn't passed a stool at

all by the time the midwife arrived on the Friday afternoon. The midwife was concerned and asked us to go to the hospital to visit a doctor. After blood tests etc., we were told Ethan was ok and that symptoms were due to the breastfeeding issues. During the hospital visit I had called my aunty to explain the situation. As much as my aunty was desperate to help out, she lived 60 miles away from where I lived and I didn't want to hassle her or ask her to travel to see me every day. I now know that she really didn't mind and wanted to help me but she didn't want to force herself on me. So I really wasn't using her experience as much as I should have. I was started to feel a failure and I didn't want her to see this. Anyway Margaret came to visit on the Friday evening and told Allan to go buy a hand expresser which he did. She advised me to express as much as possible whilst still trying with Ethan, and so if he wasn't able to latch on properly to cup feed him some expressed milk. Margaret gave me some hints and tips to try e.g. to use the pump before I tried to feed Ethan to help harden my nipple. With the advice from Margaret and the support from the daily midwifes I continued to try and bf Ethan. I was successfully feeding at times, I was pumping my nipple,

I was expressing milk and finally Ethan was starting to put on some weight. Things were starting to look good and then....my nipples became cracked....Ouch! For me this pain was worse than labour. I remember crying one night with the pain when feeding Ethan in bed. I remember having to pump for a whole day to try and give my nipples some breathing space....I managed this for three weeks and then I started to resent feeding my baby. I started to dread him waking for his feeds....this was not how I imagined. Margaret told me things would get easier through time, but I just couldn't see the light at the end of the tunnel and I didn't want this interfering with my relationship with my son. I thought bf was supposed to bring a closer bond with your baby? Not in my case! I then made the hardest decision to introduce formula to Ethan after a month. I managed to express for a further two weeks however as the days went pass I was expressing less volume until this volume became less than an oz. each . I made the decision to stop feeding my son breast milk. I felt a failure, I didn't contact my aunt for two weeks and I couldn't stop crying. I finally came to terms with my decision and the reasons why I had chosen this path. I do still believe breast is best and this experience won't stop me trying again in the future. However, my nipples have now become inverted after bf (has anyone else experienced this?) and I'm worried it may cause similar - if not more challenges next time round. Hopefully not!!

So in summary – despite what could have been, with the meconium, the back to back baby and not being able to have my water birth, I had a very positive first birth experience. I am disappointed in my breast feeding experience however I hope to be successful next time round. My baby boy is healthy and happy and is loved very much and to me that is all that matters <3

Tools for birth: What's in your tool bag?

Natural Comfort Measures for Birth:

Comfort measures are probably not going to mean that you have an entirely pain free birth. They can help minimize any discomfort though and give you a focus to help you manage any pain, keeping it at a level that you can continue without medication.

To use birth tools effectively, you must have completed the preparatory work of:

1. Being honest with yourself and your partner;

2. Identifying and releasing your fears;

3. Truly knowing and understanding who you are and what comforts you in everyday life.

Once you have a good understanding of 'how you operate' then you will be able to better identify the things that may comfort you during birth. A Birth ROCKS Mentor will be able to work through and recognise your individual coping style and recommend which tools will be most likely to work for you.

There are four main different types of comfort measures used while birthing. Depending on your everyday coping style, some of these will be better suited to your needs and senses than others.

What kinds of things can comfort me during birth? The 4 P's

1. Changing **Positions** and making sure that you that move around during birth are important because you can change the location of the pressure and help your baby to move further along the birth path. It can also help to speed up labour. Have a think about what your birth partner can do to help with regards to positions.

Assisting in you in changing position can be an important part of their role.

This is where your pregnancy yoga practice comes into play. I'm not suggesting you dive into a headstand but the strengthening of the legs for example, can be great for helping you to remain mobile and to assume positions such as squatting and all fours.

You might think that you'll be most comfortable lying on the bed, perhaps because you've seen lots of women in labour on the TV doing so. However, keeping as upright as you can help to speed up your labour and will make your better able to move and be comfortable. Even if you are lying on the bed, try not to lie completely flat, prop your hips up with some pillows or sit slightly upright.

Positions to consider during birthing

Staying upright makes the best use of gravity and is generally easier to prepare baby for exit. Upright positions can help lessen any discomfort during surges and make it easier for your birth partner to massage your back or to help you move around.

- Leaning onto a birth ball or chair offers support or put your arms round your partner's neck or waist and lean on them.

- Try kneeling on a beanbag or cushion and then lean forwards onto a chair.

- You can also try leaning onto the bed or a window to get the added advantage of getting plenty of fresh air.

- Go onto all fours and try some cat curls or swaying your hips backwards and forwards.

- Sit astride a chair, resting your head on a pillow on top of the chair back.

- Try toilet sitting, lean forwards, or try sitting astride the toilet, with your head resting on the cistern. This was a personal favourite of mine during labour. Toilet sitting has the added advantage of allowing the body to relax and open naturally. When we sit on the loo, the sphincter relaxes and releases as we do when our bowels move. By sitting on the toilet, we encourage the cervix to do the same.

2. **Props** are simple physical props you can keep in your 'tool bag.' Your tool kit could include things like wooden spoons, heat packs or even fancy birth-kit, like a TENS machine.

Things you can find at home: Using a tennis ball during labour

Because of its size and texture of a tennis ball, it makes it a great massage tool during labour. Any soft ball will do, it doesn't have to be for tennis.

You can use a tennis ball to evenly distribute the pressure during a massage. Have your birth partner place the ball on your lower back and ask them to roll the ball in small circles. Another option is to lean into the ball against the wall. Place the tennis ball at your lower back so that it provides pressure as you lean on the wall. You can move to roll the ball around or provide more pressure where and when you need it. This feels awesome, even if you are not in labour and it's brilliant for relieving pregnancy related lower back pain.

3. **Peace** or Relaxation is essential for natural childbirth as we talked about earlier, if we are relaxed, we won't be tense and if we are not tense, we minimize pain. Relaxation techniques such as self-hypnosis, yoga and yogic breathing, deep relaxation, visualization and vocalization are fantastic peace inducing practices.

The Full YogaBellies Breath: This is one of the breathing techniques I teach to my prenatal yoga and Birth ROCKS mums for releasing tension during pregnancy and birth. This is a great technique proven to lower blood pressure, relieve insomnia and make you feel generally calmer, happier and A-OK.

You can use FYB during pregnancy during the day or last thing at night to help to chill and get to sleep. This breathing technique is also used during the first part of labour to help you relax, get in the zone and release any tension that may have built up in the body during contractions.

Take a deep inhale through the nose, become aware of the turn of the breath, and then allow a deep exhale through the nose. Try to make sure the exhale is about twice as long as the inhale, so really releasing on the exhale.

You can count in for 3 and out for 6, in for 2 and out for 4 etc. Make the breath as short or as long as you need to be comfortable. Do not force the breath and at the end of the exhale, just gently allow it to turn back into an inhale.

Just bring your attention to the breath. Become aware of the cool inhale through the nose, the turn of the breath, and the warm exhale through the nose. On the exhale, just let it all out. Let it go.

Allow the muscles of the face and the jaw to relax. Allow a smile to form on the face allowing the back of the throat to open up for deeper breathing. And relax. It's as simple as that, just use the breath to RELEASE.

4. **Pamper** or Touch and Massage are fantastic if you like to 'feel' relaxation. Massage and touch therapies such as acupressure, acupuncture and reflexology work to minimize pain and tension and help to release energy during labour. You can also add in aromatherapy oils which can offer additional benefits to labouring mums.

Massage during Labour

Women all feel differently about massage during the stages of birthing. Women in labour generally do not want to be touched after contractions have begun. Being touched during labour when you don't want to be touched can be really distracting and upsetting so agree a 'signal' with your partner that they understand as touch me/don't touch me.

Your birth partner should probably wait until the surge is over and then ask you when you would most like a massage. The areas of the body that you will probably enjoy having massaged during labour include the back, the buttocks and bum, thighs, legs, tummy and hands. Reflexology on the feet can be very pleasant also. Keep in mind that not everyone wants to be touched during labour. Mum should change massage positions until she finds one that is comfortable for her.

The Birth of Baby Simone

Mum Kate Kleyn, living in Cyprus found out she was pregnant age 23 with her fist baby Simone. Kate had a natural birth despite a seventy per cent caesarean section rate in Cyprus.

When I fell pregnant with Simone I was 23 years old, just moved out of my mom and dad's house with my fiancé of 8 years and we were starting a new life together, becoming independent.

I was working at a lawyer's office at the time and found out that I was pregnant on New Year's Eve. I started feeling a little queasy for a few weeks before and there was no sign of my period, I kept denying that there was any possibility that I was pregnant, as I have had irregular periods in the past. My breasts started to hurt as well and I kept saying to myself: <my period is coming I know it>. On New Year's Eve 2008, we went to a party after work during lunch time and we all went in my boss's car, the whole way there I felt really sick.

When we arrived we dished up and sat down to eat, I couldn't really eat and some of the smells were making me feel nauseous. I remember I excused myself from the table and went to the toilet, were I vomited and then washed my hands and face and looked at myself in the mirror <You are soooo pregnant Kate>, I said to myself, I had finally accepted that this could be possible. When I looked into my eyes I saw me but I also saw another soul, it was a very strange experience, I somehow knew that someone else was inside of me, another little pure soul!

My dad was sitting on the opposite table from where I was sitting and all I kept thinking was <Oh! My god how am I going to tell my parents that I am pregnant? Being the oldest in the family and had just started my life being independent and finding out that I was pregnant was just crazy! Everything was happening really fast! However I went back outside and just couldn't wait to get home to my hubby and go and lay down... I felt so sick and tired... I just kept looking at my dad, waving at him and saying to myself: < You are sooo going to be a grandfather>!!

Later on we left and I got into my car and started driving off to go home. When I arrived home I just went to bed to lie down because I just felt so ill. My husband was stressed out and adamant to go and get a pregnancy test! I was still in denial. After a lot of conversing he convinced me to go, as long as I don't see the results :)

So, off we went on an adventure to purchase a pregnancy test. Now on New Year's Eve to find a pharmacy that's open in Paphos is a bit difficult, but we did find one and went home.

I took the test and off I ran into my room, my husband sat waiting for the result, and when he saw it he just looked at me and ran into the kitchen to pour a glass of whiskey! I knew straight away just by his look that I was pregnant and now it was official. I didn't tell anyone, I kept it to myself until I confirmed it with the doctor, however I did tell my sister, who came with me to the doctor for support.

It was New Year's Eve and I went to bed at 10:00, while my husband stayed up to welcome the New Year with his brother, I felt so ill that I couldn't stay up.

My pregnancy with Simone ran very smoothly, apart from my morning sickness that lasted until 12 weeks, which was horrible. I carried on working at the lawyer's office. After my first trimester, I started Yoga classes which really helped me focus and relax. I tried to go every day and on the days that I couldn't make it, I would practice at home. I had done Yoga before, so I knew quite a bit about it. Meditating and bonding with my unborn baby was just amazing. My Yoga teacher was great! I was the only pregnant lady in the class and she looked after me, she sometimes would play some hemi -sync music, which is said to stimulate the brain in different ways, Simone used to kick around like crazy when she used to hear it! I carried on doing Yoga until 37 weeks. Now I was due in August and believe me it is really hot in Cyprus during the summer time, how I did it I don't know!

When summer started I also began swimming in the sea every day! It was so nice, a lot of people used to think that I was crazy. They used to look at me really strange, as if they have never seen a pregnant woman on the beach or something, as if it was gross! I didn't care, I loved my body and my baby and I loved being pregnant! I made sure that I ate very healthily too.

Sometime during July, I took early leave from work and started my maternity leave too, as it was too hot and I was getting big! I and my husband decided to get married as well, just a small little wedding. It was so strange.... The year 2009 was the year of the OX, which I am and so is Simone as she was born that year. We got married on the 24th of July, Simone was born on the 24th of August and a week later I turned 24! It was indeed the luckiest and best year of my life :)

The last week of pregnancy I was getting really big and tired, but still carried on swimming and doing my Yoga and walking a lot! On the 23rd of August me and my husband went to the beach, were we spent to whole day there, it was so nice, he dared me to swim up to the boyes (balls) and back. I remember saying to him< are you crazy?>, but I did it! I swam all the way there and all the way back! My Braxton hicks started becoming a little more intense, so we decided to go home to relax.

Than night, I started taking my homeopathic remedies and drinking my teas. Something inside of me said <get your sterilizer out and sterilize your bottles and stuff> I did and then we went to bed as we had a long and tiring day! I'm sure that big swim helped me go into labour.

At around 4:30 in the morning I woke up in bed with water leaking, I thought I had peed, but couldn't be bothered to get up. Then another gush of water and I got up to go to the toilet. As I sat on the toilet some more water came out and I had some blood! I knew the baby was coming.... I took a deep breath and calmly walked back into the room. My husband was still sleeping, all I did was nudge him softly and he jumped out of bed and shouted < the baby is coming!!>. It's as if he knew, he felt it, I told him to relax and calmly just call the doctor to see what we shall do. The doctor told us to leave and head for the clinic and he would be there around 6:00am. So we got our gear and started to head down to the clinic, being a first baby and not having much experience, we didn't know what to expect.

When we arrived at the clinic, my water kept gushing and my rushes were getting a little stronger and longer. I was sent upstairs, where the nurses put me in my room and gave me and I.V and an enema. I wanted to walk around which I did for a while and then the doctor came to check me, I was still only 2cm dilated, he told me that I would give birth around 6pm. I sat calmly in my bed as my rushes were not very strong and just occasionally getting up and walking around. Around 12, my rushes felt really strong and I was really feeling them now! I kept walking around and felt the urge to sit on the toilet. Next to the toilet there was a heating rail for the towels which I kept holding on to and squeezing it, I remember my husband telling me that I nearly pulled it off the wall.

My husband was very supportive, but he was also panicking a little and didn't really know what to do for me, so I just told him not to worry and just let me be! He did and that helped the situation a lot!

I felt very psychedelic and high, I was in a trance, the doctor and the nurses kept on coming in and out the room, I felt a little violated with them looking at me and hovering around me, I don't think they had a lot of natural births, so it was quite a big thing for them to see. Most of the women have caesareans in my Country. Me, I chose a natural, drug free birth, which was awesome , but at the time I did find myself screaming for drugs, I believe that this was during transition, at this point my mother came and she held my hand and helped me through it. The doctor came at 1:15 pm to check me, I was around 5-6cm dilated and he told me that I have a long way to go yet. So he left and he told my husband that I would have the baby later on in the afternoon and that he was on his way to go and have lunch.

My husband came back into the room and I wanted that baby out right now, so I squatted and imagined her coming through. My rushes were very strong now and I felt very alert of my surroundings, I suddenly felt and said: <I need to push>. My husband just looked at me and I said to him, "Go and call someone, I need to push now!" He went to call the doctor and a nurse came in to put my on a wheel chair to take me downstairs to the delivery room. This procedure is very wrong I believe, because it is very difficult for a woman to just hop onto a wheelchair while she is in transition, taken into an elevator and then be flipped onto a bed in the delivery room.

The doctor came rushing into the delivery room and he said to me, "That was quick." I remember being put on the delivery bed and I was holding my husband's hand really tight, I would not let him go, the nurse and the doctor were telling me when to push, but I knew myself when to push, I pushed my baby out in three big pushes, it was an amazing and ecstatic feeling! Simone Angel Kleyn born on the 24/08/2009, @ 1:32pm weighing 2,800kg. As soon as I saw her I just started crying out loud < my baby, our baby>, I wanted her now to hold her and cuddle her, but the doctor took her to the other side of the room, quickly checked her and then gave her to me in my arms! She was born with her eyes wide open, staring into this world and looking around, as if she was looking for her parents! The feeling was amazing, to be looked at by this beautiful soul in such a way as if she was saying hi mom and dad, I'm here, I'm glad to be here with you. Me and my husband were holding her and loving her together as a family while I delivered the placenta and the doctor stitched me up.

My family was outside the delivery room waiting, and when we finished they took us back to my room, where I was given my child to breastfeed and bond with. Later in the afternoon I had many more visitors, friends and family. I couldn't believe that I had become a mother. The feeling was absolutely amazing and scary at the same time, I was afraid to go home; I didn't know what to do or how to do it. I knew deep down inside of me that my mother's instinct would kick in eventually and that I would soon get into it.

The clinic were very nice to us, they let my husband stay with me in my room in the other bed overnight and didn't charge us extra for it. During this time we both sat in the room with our baby, admiring her. There was so much love that filled the room and the bond was very strong.

Why Yoga Makes Mummies Happy

The role of Yoga in creating the love hormone 'Oxytocin'

Now it would be just plain wrong of me to ignore the opportunity to introduce you to yoga during pregnancy when we are talking about tools for pregnancy and birth. The fact is that yoga actually makes you happier. The 'love hormone' Oxytocin helps you to relax and reduces blood pressure and cortisol levels. Yoga is now well recognised as one of the ways to encourage the body to release this amazing hormone and built in anti-stress mechanism.

When the various limbs of yoga are practised, oxytocin is released. Deep breathing warms the body, and warmth is one of the key elements that allow us to release Oxytocin. By taking the body through the practice of yoga asana (postures) we warm the muscles and joints, make the physical body more comfortable and relaxed. By then continuing the practice with savasana (deep relaxation) and meditation, we encourage the production of oxytocin even further.

What is Oxytocin?

Oxytocin is that magical hormone that rushes through the body when we first fall in love. Oxytocin can take us to the dizzy heights of a love sickness that makes food and sleep seem so much less important than looking into the eyes of our new found love.

Some of oxytocin's main functions are preparing the female body for childbirth, stimulating milk production and 'let down' so that baby can nurse, and encouraging the bond between mum and her new-born baby.

The hormone is also plays an important part in sexual arousal and is released when you have an orgasm. It's important in nonsexual relationships too and presence of the hormone has shown to increase trust, generosity, and cooperation. It can also create a nurturing aspect within males and females who are not parents.

Why does Yoga make you happy?

Yogic breathing (of course!) When the vagus nerve is inflamed your breathing becomes shallower. Your body has gone into fight or flight mode and you have started to panic. Stop right here and allow yourself to breathe deeply. Pranayama (or yogic breathing) encourages taking time to just stop, and focus on the breath.

Pregnancy and motherhood can bring a lot of huge physical, emotional and environmental changes that can be difficult to adapt to. Taking some time each week to just BREATHE during yoga class, bringing your attention to the breath, focusing on the breath alone, not worrying about anything else, can allow oxytocin to be released and deepen that relaxation. Slow steady breathing is all that you need. Sometimes we get so caught up in 'getting the posture' that we forget to breathe. Check yourself and make sure you ARE actually breathing (you'd be surprised.)

Warming the body through the practice of Asana

It is important to warm the body before undertaking the physical practice of yoga (asana) so as not to damage any joints and to ease the body gently into the postures. This is especially important for pregnant and post natal women, whose bodies are and have undergone physical stress and growth over a period of time. During the practice of asana and pranayama, the body generates heat and warms the body inside and out. Extra bonus? When we are warm and relaxed, the body releases more oxytocin...

Chilling in Savasana

At the end of class, don't just jump up and run out of class. Savasana, deep relaxation at the end of class is your reward for all of your hard effort earlier on. Learn to enjoy the relaxation, be aware of any random thoughts that go through your mind – and just let them go. This is known as 'monkey mind' (What will I have for dinner? What did she mean by that?) Acknowledge these meaningless thoughts and really take time for yourself – just focus on the life force – the breath. That's all you need to do. And enjoy the scrummy feeling of the copious oxytocin rushing through your body. Sigh.

Why is Oxytocin so important for mummies?

In a study of 65 women with depression and anxiety, the 34 women who took a yoga class twice a week for two months showed a significant decrease in depression and anxiety symptoms, compared to the 31 women who were not in the class.

During Birth

Oxytocin helps birthing women through labour encouraging surges or contractions as well as providing pain relieving endorphins and an altered state of consciousness or bliss (known as labour land) that makes most of childbirth seems 'dream like' or surreal. As soon as baby is born, it makes mum fall in love in the greatest way possible, with their new-born baby.

In the first few moments after giving birth, a mother receives the largest rush of oxytocin that she will ever experience in her lifetime. Oxytocin flows between mother and child every time baby is breastfed which encourages bonding and attachment.

During birth we can encourage the release of oxytocin by making sure that mum has privacy, feels safe and comfortable, has a dimmed room and is left in peace. Yogic breathing and practice of adapted savasana during childbirth can aid the release of this special hormone.

Antenatal and Postnatal Depression

Yoga helps to balance hormones and stabilizes the endocrine system. By practising yogic relaxation techniques, we can balance cortical activities and the nervous and endocrine systems, reducing the body's reaction to stress. As a result, the body produces less adrenaline, noradrenaline and cortisol, (all stress hormones) and mum feels much more balanced and stress free.

Also, prenatal depression studies indicate clinical depression alleviates by half if only we can talk to a friend who listens to us and oxytocin is shown to increase when we receive empathy. The social aspects of getting out to perinatal yoga classes either before or with baby help mum and baby socialize with other mums around them.

Baby Bonding

Remember oxytocin is about being personal in ways that give our time together significance and shape moments of laughter and pleasure. Follow the instinct to reach out and strengthen ties with invitations to share together and enjoy your pregnancy and life.

There is ample evidence, that **oxytocin** and another hormone known as **vasopressin** are critical for the bonding process, especially as it relates to social and reproductive behaviour. Both chemicals help encourage bonding and maternal behaviour.

Yoga for Pregnancy and Birth

"I don't practice yoga," I hear you say. "It's not my bag. It's too hippy dippy for me. I'd much rather go for a run."

Okay well don't knock it just yet. I'm not going to bang on about it, but did you know that everything we do is actually yoga?

Yoga is....

Now here are ten little bits of interesting information that you probably didn't know about yoga, which just might encourage you to think again.

10 things you didn't know about yoga during pregnancy

As much as you may have wanted to become pregnant, it can still create a number of conflicting emotions when those two little lines appear on the pregnancy test. Practicing yoga during pregnancy can help you work through these emotions and help you stay healthy.

Yoga in pregnancy helps you maintain your flexibility and health. It can also help you to become positive about birth and parenting. Here are some things you probably didn't know about yoga for pregnancy and birth.

Yoga is not a cult!

People have lots of preconceived ideas about what yoga is and who 'should' practice it. Anyone can do yoga, it helps you become flexible and calm so don't be put off by serene looking photos of people with their legs around their neck! Perinatal yoga is gentle and the focus is about turning inward and connecting with baby while staying fit, flexible and calm.

Your choice of teacher is vital to your safety

It's important to find a yoga teacher that's right for you especially if you're new to yoga. Look for a yoga teacher that can cater for all levels and make you feel comfortable wherever you are in your pregnancy or your yoga journey. It is important to attend a class with a fully qualified teacher for pregnant women accredited by Yoga Alliance or the IYN. If you're prospective teacher does not hold a reputable Perinatal Yoga Teacher Training qualification look elsewhere!

You don't need to be able to stand on your head

Don't worry if you've never tried yoga before. It's very likely that the rest of the class will have done very little or no yoga at all before attending. Your pregnancy yoga teacher will set a steady pace. The focus is on practising at the level you feel comfortable at – everyone will be at a different stage of pregnancy and feel differently so it's important to focus on what feels best for you (and baby.)

It's about listening to your body and your baby

The most important thing is not to force yourself (or baby) to do anything you don't feel comfortable with. It's important to listen to your body's signals and slow down, even if you had a regular dynamic yoga practice before pregnancy.

You can allow yourself to slow down

If you have practised yoga before or perhaps have been a dedicated runner or gymnast, prenatal yoga can help you come to terms with the fact that it's no longer just about you! Super fit mums can often find it hard to slow down during pregnancy, but this is just as important as keeping fit. Realizing that you can't do everything the way you used to before you were pregnant is the first lesson in being a parent.

Pranayama (yogic breathing) will be a big part of your pregnancy yoga class. This has been shown to lower blood pressure, help you sleep at night and relax during labour.

Yoga can help you prepare for labour and birth

A pregnancy yoga class isn't just about keeping fit. As well as, especially adapted yoga postures which are safe and beneficial during pregnancy, pregnancy yoga helps you to learn breathing techniques to use to calm and soothe the mind. These can be used during pregnancy, birth and beyond.

Yoga can help get baby into the correct position

During the pregnancy yoga class your teacher will lead discussions on useful postures to help get baby into the correct position for birth and to help turn a breech baby.

You will learn about positions for birth

Your teacher will look at postures and positions you can assume during labour and birth to assist baby's easy entry into the world. Your yoga teacher will be able to advise you on which postures are best suited to any specific conditions that you may be suffering from as a result of pregnancy, such as pelvic girdle pain.

You can enjoy relaxation and self-hypnosis

At the end of class, pregnancy yoga often includes a deep relaxation (savasana) and self-hypnosis session, which practised regularly helps mum remain calm and positive about pregnancy and birth. And yes, we do have lots of sleeping mummies during this part!

You will get to meet like-minded mummies

Pregnancy yoga classes are the perfect place to meet other likeminded mummies. It's so important to meet other mums locally who are at the same stage in life as you and going through the same thing. Peer support will help you through the ups and downs of pregnancy and parenthood and reassure you that you and your baby are 'normal' and that someone else has probably had the same issue.

Five easy yoga postures to get you started with Yoga during Pregnancy

Here are five easy to try yoga postures to do at home. Remember that unless you are an experienced yoga practitioner with an existing practice, you should not undertake yoga until 14-16 weeks gestation. I highly recommend if you are completely new to yoga, then you should join a special prenatal yoga class.

Cat Curls (Bidalasana): Bidalasana helps relieve lower back pain and to release the length of the spine, a common problem during pregnancy. Get down on your hands and knees with hands placed directly under shoulders and knees under the hips.

Inhale and lift your heart, stretch back through your tail and concave your spine.

Exhale and roll your spine, lowering the head, pressing through the hands back to straight back. Cat Curls in pregnancy differ from your normal cat curl as we don't curl the abdomen towards the floor, after curling up we simply return to flat back or table top. Repeat following your breath – Inhale as your curl the spine up and exhale back to flat back.

Childs Pose (Balasana): From any kneeling position, sit your tail back toward your heels. Take the knees as far apart as you need to make your bump comfortable. Sit back as far as is comfortable and rest your head toward the mat. If you can't reach your head to the mat, rest your chin on your hands. You can stack your fists and rest your forehead there or use a block if you can't quite get down. Otherwise, you can stretch your arms out long in front of you and lower your head all the way to the mat. Avoid balasana if suffering from sciatica.

Bound Angle Pose (Baddha Konasana) Baddha Konasana is a classic pregnancy yoga posture and is excellent for helping to open up the hips and pelvis in preparation for birth. This is a posture that be practised at night while reading a book or watching TV and is especially important for the later stages of pregnancy in the third trimester.

Sit on your mat with the soles of the feet together. Bring your heels as close to the groin as possible and pull the shoulder back and down away from the ears to straighten the spine. Hold the feet with the hands and (with a straight spine) begin to gently bend forwards from the hips – only as much as is comfortable – please do not squish your baby! Remember to breathe in and out through the nose.

Downward Facing Dog (Adho Mukkha Svanasana): Downward dog can be practised with feet wider apart than normal to accommodate your bump, although ideally no further apart than hip width.

Push into the palms of the hands and pull up on the hip bones. When and if ready, takes the heels to the mat. It's fine to keep the knees bent when pregnant. Focus on stretching from the hands to hips, lengthening the back. Only hold any inversion for 5 seconds during pregnancy and if you feel dizzy or nauseous at all, come back down onto the mat and into child pose and relax.

Yoga Squats (Malasana): Squats are great for building strength and stamina during pregnancy and in preparation for birth. Many women like to squat while birthing. As you get bigger in pregnancy, use props such as blocks, bolsters or a rolled up blanket to rest your bottom on. Focus on relaxing and letting your breath drop deeply into your belly. Stand facing the back of a chair with your feet slightly wider than hip-width apart, toes pointed outward. Squat down toward the floor as though you were going to sit down in a chair. Contract the abdominal muscles, lift your chest, and pull the shoulders back and down. Most of your weight should be toward your heels. This can be done against the wall for support. Remember to avoid wide legged postures if suffering from pelvic girdle pain or PSD.

Nicola McConville's Birth Story,

First time mum to baby Johnny in Munich, Germany

I had a wonderful and easy pregnancy and decided that I didn't need to know anything about childbirth. I was feeling positive and that was enough. It would go down exactly as it should; a slow build-up of contractions then the calm controlled final stage of labour of pushing the baby out. I didn't want anything to scare me or change that. I felt under pressure to have a birth plan, since I have a plan for everything else in life, but it was basic and it simply stated no drugs, no C-section and no episiotomy (unless absolutely necessary), if only such requests could easily be honoured! In actual fact I did accomplish the first two but quickly realised that you can't plan a birth in this way.

The best advice that I got was from Cheryl MacDonald, my dear friend and author of this book. She told me about Birth ROCKS concepts, but since I lived far away I unfortunately couldn't participate, but a few simple words went a long way in helping me through my birth. She taught me that everyone manages pain and childbirth in their own unique way and the best way to prepare would be to get to know myself. I thought to myself how on earth can I possibly do that until I am in the situation, but she guided me to discuss painful events in my life and think about how I dealt with them. The first thing that sprang to mind was getting my tattoo. For some it is just a scratch, for me it was unimaginable pain. That taught me my first lesson, everyone reacts to everything differently. I could run marathons, do triathlons, fast for a week, get body piercings, but not a tattoo!

Cheryl asked me to tune into how exactly I felt at that moment and I remembered being unusually silent, crying on the inside with wet tears in my eyes and almost holding my breath whilst trying to hold onto my strength and perseverance. Would you believe that my childbirth was exactly that? It couldn't have been more exact. I did not utter one word, not even when asked a question.

My labour shocked me to the core. It was fast and furious! Less than 2 hours and too fast for medication or even my hospital gown! Not at all how I had planned or foreseen. The only thing that kept me calm was knowing that I was reacting exactly the way we had discussed, which gave me the feeling that I was somehow, through all the chaos, in control.

Like so many mums, although my birth was perfect on paper and actually perfect to the outside world (My husband said that I made it look easy!) I suffered mentally afterwards because it was not what I had planned. I had imagined a slow build up with me totally in control, not a sudden onset directly to active labour and a baby less than two hours later. The best birth preparation that I actually did was to listen to Cheryl guide me to get to know myself and how I handled pain, not to imagine how it will look, how long it will be or how I thought it would feel.

Not only was I in shock that I wasn't dressed, or that it happened so fast, for me it felt so different than I imagined or how it felt for other women. The contraction pain for me was manageable, but my body was weak from the fast and hard contractions and the nausea was so strong. I was not at all prepared for that and it caused panic and fear. I could not have prepared for that because everyone woman is different and that is why expecting the unexpected without a predetermined picture is very important, something I failed to understand. I was right in not having a too detailed plan but sub consciously I had managed to picture how I expected it to go, either from media or other mothers. But fortunately for me the calm in the storm was suddenly realising Cheryl was right, I am acting the way we discussed. A-ha suddenly a known in this unknown mess and that is what I held onto throughout the birth and beyond. That is what got me through. Even in the post birth guilt phase of the birth not going exactly to plan, I still took great comfort from the fact that I was able to determine my reaction beforehand. Thus if I were to go through it again, I would focus on getting to know me and not predicting how it will go or feel. Even having gone through childbirth, the next could be totally different!

What about drugs?

Yep, drugs are also an option. As I said at the beginning of the book, the purpose of this book is not to preach about what you should or shouldn't do during birth, but to get you thinking about what you want – and don't want – from childbirth and how to best go about achieving that outcome.

I'm not going to list all of the drugs and interventions available but instead give you a quick overview of why natural birth is:

1. Safer for you and baby;
2. A faster birth than when than having drugs;
3. Has less post-partum recovery time afterwards

The main thing is to actually have the correct information. So I want to provide you some information on why, top line, drugs are not always the easiest option. If you want to find out more about drugs and their pros and cons, then you'll have to buy another book, sorry ☺

Natural Birth Benefit 1: Its safer for you and your baby

Since there are no epidurals or other drugs administered to the mother, natural childbirth removes the dangers of possible toxics which may come in contact with the baby. There are some cases where anaesthesia does more harm than good to both mother and baby.

In addition, forceps applied to pull out the baby from the mother's birth canal are notorious for the hazards they may bring. Most of the time forceps leave marks on the baby's soft forehead or even some cases cause brain damage. An epidural prevents the mother from feeling if she is pushing correctly, so forceps may be used to help the mother's push. With natural childbirth, the mother knows that the baby is going out well, and there is usually no need for forceps.

Babies birthed without drugs tend to bond more quickly with their mum. The babies tend to be able to use their instincts better, and are generally more responsive to their parents touch.

Natural Birth Benefit 2: Natural Childbirth is Faster

Need I go any further? Using drugs such as an epidural prevents mum from feeling – anything – below the waist. So you can't feel as baby progresses or when you need to push. This can lead to excessive tearing of the perineum. Ultimately, the whole process will be faster when compared to being under anaesthesia.

Breathing through your surges or contractions is more effective when no sedatives have been given, as you can feel what you are doing. There are no risks of side effects for mum and baby when no anaesthesia has been administered. For example, if mum has pethidine, did you know that this can make baby sleepy and dazed, less likely to take to the breast and less successful at feeding all round.

Natural Birth Benefit 3: It takes less time to recover

Mums who have had a natural birth heal quicker than those who have given birth using drugs. They don't need to lie down (as is the case with an epidural) and will be able to move around and make themselves comfortable during birthing. They won't be groggy from the drugs which mean they will be better able to experience the first moments of their babies' lives: why would you want to miss this??

Mums birthing in hospitals tend to stay shorter periods of time and can get back to their normal activities after a couple of days. The healing process is also shorter, and mums generally feel more connected to their new baby.

But what if I decide I want drugs anyway?

If you have read the information above and still feel strongly that you want to have drugs during childbirth, then that's okay. We want women to feel empowered and supported and if considering everything we've just talked about, you still feel that drugs will do this for you, then absolutely have drugs during the birth. But you need to be aware (I said we would be honest with you) that the drugs don't work and they don't make it easier.

I remember people saying to me when I mentioned that I wanted to have a natural birth, "Why are you being a martyr? Just have an epidural. It's great you won't feel anything!" I don't want anyone to be a martyr or to be in pain, I just want you to know that there are honestly more comfortable, easier and more effective natural ways of dealing with the sensations of childbirth than drugs.

The body's natural pain killers: Endorphins

Our body has an AMAZING natural pain killer built in called endorphins. That's why we don't need artificial drugs!

A woman's body produces *beta-endorphins* that are opiate-like substances to counter the pain of the surges or contractions of childbirth. The levels of endorphins rise as the labour progresses – literally to match the increasing intensity of the contractions. Isn't this amazing??

So if we have an epidural for example, the endorphins switch off. The artificial medication takes the place of our natural pain killers, the endorphins. So if an epidural is allowed to "wear off" for the second stage of labour, to allow mums to breathe baby down or push, mum will only have the endorphin level of earlier in labour. It will not have increased with the strength of the surges as it would have done had she chosen not to have artificial drugs. So in fact mum will be in pain as her body's natural defences will not be at their peak.

Should I be induced?

In theory, Induction sounds like a great idea. You've made it to 39 weeks of labour and you are tired. You struggle to fit through doors, 'tired' doesn't even touch your exhaustion levels, you haven't seen your feet in weeks and frankly, you'd like to just have your baby now thank you.

Many people choose to have inductions for social reasons (I'm a bridesmaid at a wedding in a few weeks and need to fit into the dress) and some people for medical reasons (pre-eclampsia for example.) If it is an actual option you are considering, then again I would ask you to be aware of some facts around induction. If you know that you will be induced for medical reasons, then that is fine and it is a fantastic tool when there is a medical necessity.

- Induction is generally brought on using powerful drugs or a device to break the waters. Both of these techniques can cause foetal distress and problems in labour which are best to be avoided if it's an option to do so. There can be a risk of increased risk of abnormal foetal heart rate, shoulder dystocia and other problems with the baby in labour.
- Be aware that as induced labour is not actually 'real' labour, it can bring on very powerful and

painful contractions. It's not an easy ride and you could find yourself in labour for a long, long time as your body has basically been forced into labour before its ready. Be patient woman, baby will come out when they are fully cooked!

- There also appears to be a higher risk of baby having to go to a neonatal until after being born as baby was not ready to arrive yet.
- There is an increased risk of C-section also as often labour induction is unsuccessful as it's often too far along to 'back out.'
- Baby can also be more likely to be jaundiced. (Information from March of Dimes 2006.)

What about C-sections?

Ah C-sections. Often seen as an easy option. You can now choose to 'book in' on your chosen date to have baby taken out at your convenience. But how 'convenient' is Caesarean section really? For mum and baby?

I am not against C-sections for medical reasons, or if mother is truly terrified of birth and this is the best option for her. I am against women being led to believe that this is an easy option. A C-section is major abdominal surgery and mothers need to be properly informed as to the risks of undertaking such surgery for them and their new-born baby.

I have a friend who had a very traumatic first birth and no amount of holistic therapy or hypnosis would have led her to birth again had C-section not been an option. And when I saw her after the birth of her second baby, relaxed (yet clearly in a lot of discomfort), I knew that this had been the best choice for her.

Some things to consider regarding C-sections:

- Like all surgery, C-sections have risk like infection, injury to blood vessels and organs, and serious bleeding.

- A C-section can also cause problems for babies, like breathing difficulties that need treatment in a new-born intensive care unit.
- Recovering after a C-section is also more difficult than after a vaginal birth.
- C-sections can also cause certain on-going problems. For example, C-sections can cause chronic pelvic pain in some women.
- Babies born by C-section are at increased risk of developing chronic childhood diseases like diabetes and asthma.

If your health care provider has recommended that you have a C-section and you feel uncomfortable with this, make sure that you find out exactly why this procedure is necessary. This is your body and your baby and you have every right to find out why this needs to happen.

Some questions you can ask about having a C-section:

- Why are you suggesting that I have a C-section?

- What are the benefits of having a C-section for me or my baby?
- What problems could arise if I still want to try for a vaginal birth?
- How likely are these problems to occur if I plan for a vaginal birth?
- Could this still happen if I have a C-section?
- What are the possible disadvantages and risks of a C-section?

Having an aware Caesarean

If you hoped for a natural birth, but circumstances dictate that a C-section is necessary, that doesn't mean you can't still have an amazing birth experience. All hope is not lost!

You can work with your health care provider to make sure your birth experience is still intimate and beautiful for you and your family.

Some changes you may consider to help make your birth lovely:

- Instigate early skin-to-skin contact, with either mum or dad to encourage early bonding.
- A slowed down birthing, allowing it to be as similar to a vaginal birth as possible.
- Think about having any partitions removed to allow you to see baby's arrival.
- Ask for any catheters or blood pressure cuff to be placed on the same arm to allow mum to hold and cuddle baby on arrival.
- Request ECG leads to be positioned on the back, to keep the chest free for skin-to-skin contact and breastfeeding.

This is a woman and family centred approach to caesarean birth making it as 'natural' as possible for all concerned and generally making it a more positive birthing experience.

It also helps with, better bonding, early feeding, and overall greater satisfaction with the birth experience.

The Birth of Nathan Logan

Lisa Logan, mum of one had a C-section after being diagnosed with pre-eclampsia.

I was 34 weeks pregnant and utterly terrified of birth. There was some doubt if my baby was breach and I went along to my antenatal check-up hoping to be referred for C-Section. It hadn't even occurred to me when I got pregnant that birth could scare me so much. My main fear was losing the plot during my labour and not being able to deliver my healthy, beautiful baby safely. I lost faith in my body and didn't listen to what millions of years of evolution told me, that my body was built for this task.

After my antenatal check the hospital referred me for a ... and I went along to my appointment half hoping my son would stay put & I'd be booked in for a C-section. The consultant pressed on my pregnant tummy a few times and when the pain got unbearable he told me that if I couldn't cope with that pain, there's no way I'd cope with labour and I was booked in for C-section in 2 weeks.

*I had a beautiful, peaceful birth & my son was born healthy & happy. But I will always feel that I copped out and I wasn't brave enough to birth **naturally.it** saddens me that I could have avoided unnecessary surgery if the hospital had talked my fears through with me & encouraged a natural birth instead of belittling my capability.*

I am now training as a birth preparation mentor so I can educate women & their partners on trying to make birth as natural as possible. Fear is the biggest factor contributing to pain in birth but with proper education, mentoring and reassurance (not a scathing obstetrician) natural birth can be peaceful & beautiful. A woman should never feel a C-section is the only choice because she's weak but if her birth does result in a C-section her birth is still valid, it is still hers.

Preparing for the Big Day

We have identified and released our fears, we know and understand our coping styles and we know what tools we have in our birthing kit.

What other things can you do to get ready? You can put together a birth plan.

What is a Birth Plan?

A birth plan is a plan of action for the big day. You will have one of these in the blue book that you receive from your midwife, where all of your antenatal visits are recorded. I tend to say, make a plan for birth, and then be prepared not to stick to it.

Don't turn up at your birth with a list of demands for the midwives. You cannot plan everything in birth so let's call it a list of 'birth preferences' instead. Think of things that you definitely would and wouldn't like for your birth. So quite big decisions you may want to think about could be, who will be at the birth? Will I have a doula? Will I birth at home? Will I birth in water?

Your doula or Birth ROCKS Mentor can help you put together your birth preferences and provide some guidelines on how to do this. It doesn't have to be 'War and Peace' and you only have to go into as much detail as you wish to. So perhaps you had an epidural with your first birth and do not want another one under any circumstances for this birth. Or you feel strongly about waiting until the umbilical cord stops pulsating before cutting it.

Try not to be too rigid in your birth plan and accept that there is every possibility that things won't go to plan. Be open to accepting medical assistance if necessary, even if you had hoped for a natural birth, the health of you and your baby are first and foremost.

The Basics when considering your birth preferences

- Where do I want to birth? Home/hospital/birth centre? Find out your options locally and pros and cons of each;
- Do I want to labour or birth in water? What does this mean?
- Do I want to try for a natural birth? If so, how am I going to manage any discomfort?
- Who will be my birth partner?

Where am I going to give birth?

This generally refers to a home, birth centre or hospital birth. These are your main options for birthing each with different considerations. This is something you will want to think about quite early on as your health care provider will need to make the necessary arrangements for you.

Find out about the location of each of these options in proximity to your home, the facilities available (for example, if you want to have a water birth, are there pools available?) and pros and cons of each option before you decide.

Creating a Birth Space

Even if you are not giving birth at home, you can still create a peaceful 'birth space' for the start of labour. You will want to stay at home as long as possible. Being at home helps you remain calm and relaxed, let's face it; we don't want to spend any more time in hospital than is necessary. Unless you are 4cm dilated, then the hospital staff will generally send you home until then.

Your birth space could be in your bedroom, bathroom, lounge, wherever you feel comfortable and safe. Dim the lights make sure it's cosy and warm and have anything around you that helps you feel at peace and relaxed. Play soft music and burn aromatherapy candles. Make it a lovely place to be.

Things you can do in the final furlong to make birthing easier

Perineal massage: massaging and toning the perineum to make sure that it doesn't tear during childbirth and 'pings' back into shape. Just like exercising your perineum.

Drink raspberry leaf tea: raspberry leaf tea has been shown to speed up the second part of labour when drank from around 28 weeks. Please refer to the label on the tea/capsules you are using as the dates advised often vary.

Yoga for strengthening and opening: Strengthening the leg muscles for squatting and strength bearing and also focusing on opening the hips and pelvis for comfortable birthing.

The Pregnancy and Birth of Vanessa Hope Kleyn.

This is the story of Kate's second baby Vanessa.

When I fell pregnant with Vanessa, I just started working at a Toy shop. The signs this time were less intense and I knew what to expect. I started having pains in my breasts and so I went to the doctors to make sure that everything was alright. Then that week I started having some weird cravings, and started feeling nauseous. I knew I was pregnant immediately this time.

I went to the doctor again and it was confirmed that I was pregnant, and there was a possibility that I was going to have twins! My nausea and vomiting with Vanessa was bad, it was actually worse than when I was pregnant with Simone.

My pregnancy with Vanessa was great, I was just a little stressed out due to finances. I started my Yoga, my swimming and walking again, I felt really great. It was easier to break the news to my family this time around as it was their second grandchild. They were quite a bit shocked at the beginning, but loved the idea.

This time around my job was more enjoyable, as I was working with children and toys, I was also not working full time, only part time, so I had lots of time to rest and to spend with my daughter, before the baby came. Simone bonded with her sister throughout the pregnancy, I made sure she talked to her and touched my belly a lot. We spoke about all the responsibilities and how things will change when her sister is born. She will be the oldest sister and will need to teach her little sister everything that she knows. She loved the idea and I knew that this would help prepare her correctly; I also knew that if I asked for her help and make her participate in almost everything she wouldn't feel jealous. I didn't want her to feel left out or that she was not important anymore. I tell my children every day that I love them and hug them as much as I can, they need this.

We had a really good summer and thank god we had a swimming pool at home, so I didn't have to run down to the beach every day in the heat like I did with Simone. It was so nice just to get up, have breakfast and just jump into the pool.

I worked up until my 37th week and had to stop because it was too hot and I was getting really heavy, Vanessa was a bigger baby and because I was a sales advisor at the shop, I hardly ever sat down, so the standing all the time was killing me, sometimes I would stand all day long for 5-6 hours. So I decided to just take the leave and stay at home to prepare myself for my birth and obviously get plenty of rest.

I would take Simone down to the beach some days because she used to like to play with the sand and then would go and visit my mom. My husband was working all day long so I didn't really see much of him. My nesting with Vanessa was absolutely crazy, I knew she would be with us soon, I cleaned everything in the house, and every single little thing was sorted out too. It was a mad moment, even when I visited family I would just start cleaning and sorting out their things. I actually couldn't stop, I had to tell myself to stop and just relax.

On the 12th of September, I felt really tired, I remember it was really hot and I woke up early, had some breakfast and took Simone and went down to my mother's house. I stayed on the couch the whole day and my Braxton Hicks were a little more intense than usual. I just stayed on my couch, eating, sleeping and reading. At least Simone was occupied, so I could just relax. By late afternoon I was having really strong pains but not regular, so I called my husband and told him that I wasn't feeling very good , He told me just to relax and I would be okay. I'm sure that I was going through early labour.

At some point around 6pm I felt like going for a long walk, which was really strange as I hadn't been walking much the last few weeks, due to the heat. So I asked Simone if she would like to take a long walk and she agreed. As we were walking the fresh clean air and the movement made me feel better, but every so often I would stop for a while because I would have a rush, each one becoming stronger and a little longer. By now I knew that this is going to happen today, but at the same time I was also denying it.

When we arrived back at my mom's house, I called the doctor to tell him what was happening and he advised me to just monitor myself and unless my rushes became stronger and were five minutes apart, not to worry. But he did have it in mind that there was a possibility that I would go into labour that night.

Having already had a baby before, I kind of knew what to expect, but I also knew that each birth is different too. I was wiser this time around and knew what I wanted and what to do.

The time was 8pm and I left from my mom's house and drove home, I was not in a very nice mood, in fact I was very upset and I went home crying. My husband was home and he was trying to find out what was wrong. I remember I was in the kitchen and was trying to cook but I was angry and kept crying, then I ran upstairs and went to go and lay down with my daughter, but my rushes started to become really heavy and I just couldn't lay down anymore.

I went back downstairs and tried to continue to cook, and as I was standing by the counter I kept going down into squatting position every time I would have a rush and just breathe it through until it would go away... but it wasn't going away... Around 11:30 my husband said to me you know Kate I think we better call the doctor, as we were both keeping track of the time and counting my rushes and they had become very regular and were around five minutes apart. So we called the doctor and told him that we were on the way. I went outside and walked barefoot around the swimming pool, holding my baby and looking at the stars and the moon, connecting and becoming one with Mother Nature, while my husband was getting all the things together. I started sitting on my birthing ball and doing breathing exercises to help the rushes and the baby to descend. This was really helpful.

We had to pass by my mom's house on the way to the clinic, since we had to drop of our angel, which was a little uncomfortable, because all I wanted to do was to get out and walk. We finally made it to the clinic, the doctor and the nurse were waiting for me, we went into the room and my rushes started to get really heavy now and I felt much spaced out. They put me on an IV, checked the baby's heartbeat and gave me an enema.

The doctor came to check me and I was only 2cm dilated! I was shocked, all that pain and only two centimetres? I told my husband to give me my homeopathy and do some acupressure that I showed him to help get my rushes more efficient and open up quicker.

The next thing the nurse came in and gave me an injection of something. At this point I was I labour land and didn't know what was going on. Within a few moments I started feeling woozy and weird... they gave me pethidine........it was awesome at the time, but I'm upset about it since I never asked for drugs and my doctor was very aware that I wanted a drug free natural pregnancy like the previous one. However they gave me the shot, without even asking me. My husband was exhausted and he just lay down for a while on the bed, to which he fell asleep, bless him. The nurses kept telling me to relax and lay down, save my energy and rest, but I didn't want to. I remember getting the baby's clothes and stuff ready on the bed and I was taking pictures of them.

I kept squatting and timing my rushes, it felt ecstatic! I was having rushes every one minute and resting only for a few seconds, I kept squatting and holding on to the IV pole and focusing on it. I will tell you one thing; I will never look at an IV the same way ever again!

My breathing was rhythmic and I really tried to keep calm and positive, the doctor came to check me at 2:20am, I was only 8cm dilated and he told me that it would take a long time to have this baby. As soon as he left I got of the bed and carried on holding onto the IV pole and squatting, as soon as I did this my water broke onto the floor and I started feeling the urge to push. I shouted loud: I need to push now! The nurse came in with the wheelchair and my husband just woke up and jumped off the bed! They tried to put me in the wheelchair but it was so difficult to get me out of the squatting position and onto it, but they did, it took both of them to lift me up.

I was transferred into the delivery room and put on the bed, I remember saying to my husband <I can't do this, it's too difficult> and he told me yes you can, I pushed and pushed, Vanessa was more difficult to push out than Simone, after four pushes though she was out, my baby! The doctor put her straight on my tummy while the cord was still intact, just a few minutes. She was the most beautiful baby in the world; I remembered immediately how I felt with Simone too. She cried, they cut the cord and the doctor made sure everything was alright, my husband went over and had the *most biggest smile on his face, constantly, he just kept looking at her in amazement and happiness, he couldn't take his eyes of her. I was feeling beautiful, holy and sacred; there was so much love in the room. They brought her over to me for a while, while the placenta was delivered and the doctor stitched me up.*

Vanessa Hope Kleyn, born on the 13/09/2012 at 2:30am, 3,350kg. The nurse that stayed with me during the birth, her name was Vanessa too, how strange? I told her that my daughter has the same name as you and she was so happy! We went back to our room, where they brought my baby and I breastfed her immediately, we stayed together in the room and she spent the night with us. It was so amazing, now all who was missing was Simone. I couldn't wait for her to meet her baby sister.

In the morning families came to visit us, Simone was so excited, she came in and she gave me a big hug and a love and she said to me < mommy I'm excited to see Vanessa>. So we brought her into the room, and her little face just lit up, she couldn't believe that that was her little sister.

I love my family and I love what we have accomplished together. We have a strong bond, we are united and our love for each other is unexplainable and unconditional! I'm sure we were all together before.

The Big Day: ROCK your Birth!

The Big Signs of Labour

Childbirth actually starts weeks before you feel your first contraction. Your body starts to prepare for birth in a range of different ways that may or may not notice. Even if you don't notice or see any of these things, they are still happening. The 'signs' of labour can be an indication that you will be about to give birth very soon, but the time scales vary greatly. For example, 'a show' can happen weeks or hours before you go into labour. The main thing to know is that things are moving in the right direction.

Warming up for labour

In the third trimester you may become aware of a tightening of the uterus, coming in irregular waves or after you have drank raspberry leaf tea. These practice surges or contractions are also known as Braxton-Hicks and are not real contractions at all. These waves are important to prepare the uterus for the upcoming labour. Think of Braxton Hicks as toning and strengthening the muscles of the Uterus in preparation for the big event, the same way you may be practising yoga to grow strong. Braxton Hicks don't hurt and often precede that start of labour. I personally didn't feel the point where the Braxton hicks became real labour.

'False Labour' is the term used to describe a period where you may actually have a number of regular Braxton hicks for a few hours at a time. False labour is still toning up and strengthening the body in preparation for giving birth.

You know it's the real thing when your contractions are around 5 minutes apart and regular. They will gradually become closer and closer and the waves more intense. If you suspect these are still Braxton-Hicks, try having something to eat or going for a walk about. If you find this changes the regularity of the surges or that they disappear, then this is just practice contractions

Leaky Boobies

You may get a fright when you notice that your breasts are secreting a thick yellow fluid. This is known as colostrum. Colostrum is what you produce before your milk 'comes in' and will be your baby's first food. Colostrum is amazingly good for your baby and has a very high concentration of protein and antibodies from your immune system, which protect your baby from illness for the first few days. It also acts as a laxative to help move the meconium (baby's first poo) out of their digestive system. The high levels of vitamins and minerals found in colostrum may also be important for protecting baby and in furthering their development. This is why everyone tells you that breast feeding is so important in those first few hours (weeks, months etc. etc.)

A Bloody Show: Eek!

It's not as bad as it sounds and it's actually a very promising sign that baby is en route. It does have an unfortunate name though. A bloody show is basically bloody mucus from your cervix which loosens and comes out as the cervix begins to thin and dilate. You may notice it when you go to the bathroom. Generally, a bloody show is a small amount of bright red blood and may contain a few small clumps, so don't be worried if you see this.

Toilet time

As the body prepares for birthing, it starts to clear itself out. This could result in mild diarrhoea, always a joy.

Simone Keenan Garner, tells about the birth of her three daughters

The most surprising thing I found out about being pregnant, was feeling so powerful, special and feminine! I really connected with each baby in the same way, with love, wonder, excitement, and a knowing that I was going to be so happy being a mother. And I am.

First labour/birth...I was naturally apprehensive. Second baby labour/birth. I was excited and happy during labour....third baby. I was completely enjoying the moments as I knew it was going to be my last....<3

It did cross my mind 'how on earth could I love another child as much as my first' on my second pregnancy, but the powerful force of love sorted that one out! Then, the third baby there was no worries at all on love.

On the first birth, I was prepared with precious words from a fabulous women, saying 'you are going to be climbing a

mountain'.....just when you think you can't climb any
further, a strength comes from within and you keep going
on your journey, knowing the end will be in sight, with
great results! She was so right, and I drew strength from
her words of wisdom during labour. Also, using the Golden
Thread breath that my yoga teacher had taught me. In the
pregnancy times, it didn't make sense to me. But during
labour I KNEW what they were getting at! And the
influence from these women carried me through all my
three labours and births.

I was very fortunate to experience three natural vaginal
births with the use of 'happy gas & air', and birthing
descent lasting only 10-20 minutes. I trusted and believed
in myself, the women who had influenced me and I gave in
to the process completely.

I felt a very strong connection with my babies, retreated
within myself and listened to my body & mind with
extrasensory/extraordinary perception! It was a very
spiritual and intimate experience.

Love pregnancy, love birth, love babies, love life. x

Talk me through labour and birth, what actually happens?

As labour progresses, your contractions will begin to last longer, become more intense and you will have less time in between the surges. These waves will help to get baby into the correct position and will help to push the baby and the amniotic sac against the cervix to stretch it around the baby's head. Your midwife may want to give you a vaginal examination to check 'how dilated you are.' but it's won't really give you any indication of how long you will be in labour. Many women dilate a lot (up to 7 or 8cm) in the first few hours and then dilation slows down or stops altogether. You will find that if you attempt to go to hospital before you are 4cm dilated, you will generally be sent home as you will not be considered to be in active labour.

Early in labour... This is a good time to relax in your birth space: have a bath, listen to soothing music or watch a funny film (the more you laugh the more endorphins you release!)

You will probably want to chat, to talk about what you are experiencing or want to carry on with whatever you happen to be doing. This is great and will be you occupied.

Eat and drink as normal. If you remain calm the body's digestive system will not arrest and you will be able to eat and drink what you like (within reason.)

If labour begins at night, try to go back to sleep. I know it's exciting, but it's best to get as much rest as you can and to save your energy.

At home, as your waves get progressively stronger and longer you may begin to wonder just where you are in labour and how much longer it will be before baby arrives. There is no exact measure of when baby will make an appearance and vaginal examinations without medical necessity often have little or no value with regards to determining this.

You know its active labour when...

You just feel that 'this is it.'

You probably won't feel the need to eat or drink as much at this stage. Try to keep your fluid intake high so that you don't become dehydrated and something like a lolly pop can be great to stop your mouth from becoming too dry.

You will begin to become engrossed in the birth, focusing and tuning into your body and the surges.

You probably won't want to speak to anyone and everything may seem a bit surreal. This is often known as 'labour land' and it feels like a lovely, fuzzy place, created by all of those amazing hormones rushing around your body and your deep breathing too.

You will also find that as your waves become more intense, you are less likely to be concerned by how you look or sound to other people. You may pee or poo during contractions and you probably won't even notice and you definitely won't care. Please don't worry about this, nobody will mention it to you afterwards and it's not a big deal, I promise.

No matter how long you find yourself in labour, there are usually consistent emotional and physical stages that most women experience. Midwives are usually very good at recognizing and identifying these signs and will guide you through them.

And when baby is ready to come out...

You will know baby is on their way down the birth path when you start to experience a fullness in the pelvic area. Some women describe it as a bearing down or a weighty feeling. Some women don't notice what is known as transition at all.

This is the point during birthing when you are completely dilated (10cm – yes WOW!) and baby is ready for exit. This part can be pretty intense with the waves often right on top of each other without a break in between. Please remember this is also the shortest part of labour, usually lasting 15 minutes to half an hour.

An important thing to remember at this point is that if birthing gets to the point where you think, "This is unbearable! I can't go on!" Then this means it's almost over! Please remind your birth partner to tell you this when you say it.

Try your best not to push until you have to. You can breathe baby down for most of the birth instead of pushing. During my birth, I think I have 3 or 4 pushes as baby's head was almost out. This allows the cervix to relax and open and lessens the chance of tearing the perineum.

Often women feel very hot or cold, sweat a lot, feel nauseous or vomit. You may shiver or shake, have hiccups, burp a lot and be just unable to feel comfortable in any position. This is also the most common time for the bag of waters to break naturally.

"I had a terrible experience first time round with my labour......waters broke and I didn't go into labour myself so I was induced 2 days later ......18 hours later I had a forceps delivery and I haemorrhaged (2 transfusions needed) Needless to say with my 2nd son I was petrified of labour. BUT this time I had the most amazing experience! I went into labour myself (6 days late and booked in to be induced) and progressed quickly at home. I arrived at the hospital at 9.45pm and baby Jude appeared into this world at 11.36pm. I did it all by myself with a little gas and air. My body told me when to push which felt amazing!! I got home the next afternoon on a total birthing high!! I can actually say I loved my labour this time!! Xx"

Tracey Lyon

Once baby arrives...

Why should I wait until the cord stops pulsing to cut it?

Several studies now suggest that new-born babies gain several benefits from waiting to cut the umbilical cord until at least two minutes after birth. This has now become the general procedure but if it's something you feel strongly about you may want to put it in your birth plan.

Waiting until the cord stops pulsating could result in better blood counts and iron levels for your baby. If the cord is cut prematurely, often baby will gasp for air and/or not receive all of the nutrients they receive from the placenta.

You've got your baby...now here comes the Placenta

Once baby has been born, the placenta is still attached inside of you. At some point after baby has arrived, the placenta will detach from the uterus and then be 'birthed' also. This is called the "3rd stage of labour" and can take a couple of minutes or up to an hour.

You will experience a few more surges (which you won't notice as you will be too busy gazing at your beautiful new baby) and then out pops the placenta. It is very dangerous for mum for any of the placenta to be left inside and if the placenta does not detach, it may have to be manually removed during surgery. Unfortunately, I had this pleasure after the birth of my son, but was just so happy and high about his arrival that I barely noticed.

Once the placenta has been expelled, the uterus contracts firmly, closing off the open blood vessels which had previously supplied the placenta. Without this wave, rapid blood loss could cause a big problem and be dangerous for mum also.

Bonding, the Blues and Baby Massage

Bonding after Birth

Now if you are anything like me, you spent most of your pregnancy checking your pregnancy phone app and reading books on pregnancy and birth: "At 9 weeks, baby is the size of a peanut and you will start to notice your rounded belly" etc.

Once baby arrives you may think to yourself, I'm not really sure what happens now? This is not a baby bible, but there are a few important things you will want to know about once baby arrives.

Bonding with baby when they first arrive is really important. Bonding is really a continuation of the relationship that began during pregnancy. The physical and chemical changes that were occurring in your body reminded you of the presence of this tiny person. Birth cements this bond and gives it reality. Now baby is actually here!

Tips for Bonding

- Put baby straight to the breast or chest for skin to skin contact if possible. This can aid the bonding process from the beginning.
- Make eye contact with your baby. Gaze at baby (as if you will actually be able to stop) and speak to them and acknowledge them as a person. Interact with baby from day one.
- Show respect for your baby and teach them respect for themselves by explaining to them exactly what is going on around them. For example, I would say to my son, "Okay wee guy, I'm going to take this nappy off now and put on a

new one, is that okay?" I would wait for him to respond and eventually, they do actually start to squeak in response so you are effectively having a conversation with them.

- Touch your baby. Loving touch is so important for new-borns and gentle stroking and practises such as baby massage are great for helping baby heal from any birth trauma and also gently eases them into the world outside of your tummy. Babies can often become overwhelmed with the barrage of sensations they experience after birth. Reassuring touch can help to ease this transition

The Baby Blues and Post Natal Depression

Most mums go through a brief period of feeling emotional and tearful after childbirth. Your body is going wild with all of those lovely hormones and sometimes after the initial excitement; you can hit the earth with a bump – known as the 'baby blues'. The blues usually start a week or so after giving birth and affects around 80 per cent of new mums. In fact the blues are so common that it is considered completely normal. Be aware that this feeling doesn't last too long important to be and is generally quite manageable with a good support network of helping hands around you.

Around 10-15 per cent of new mums go on to develop a more concerning and longer term depression known as postnatal depression (PND). It usually develops within six weeks of giving birth and begins gradually or comes on all of a sudden. It can range from being relatively mild to very severe.

You need to remember that if you experience the baby blues or even if PND develops, that there is help at hand. Be aware of how you are feeling and seek help. Often mums just need someone to talk to as it is such a huge change to your life

Common signs of postnatal depression

- Exhausted but can't sleep

- Lack concentration

- Feeling sad and low

- Crying for no apparent reason

- Feeling hopeless or helpless

- Feeling unable to cope

- Becoming irritable and angry

- Feeling guilty

- Becoming hostile or indifferent to your partner or baby

Overcoming PND

Be honest about how you are feeling and speak to someone. Ask for help when you need it. Try to get out of the house at least once per day. Even if it means getting baby in to the buggy and going to the shops. Fresh air and a new environment will help you feel more in touch with the rest of the world.

Meet other mums in your area. You may be the first of your friends to have a baby and this can be very lonely. Go to mum and baby classes such as baby massage (studies have shown baby massage improved the mother-baby bond and helps you interpret baby's cries.)

Consider post natal mum and baby yoga too. You can start practising gentle yoga 6-8 weeks after a normal birth and 8-10 weeks after a C-section. Be guided by how you feel and always listen to your body. Post natal yoga can help alleviate the symptoms of PND (remember all of that Oxytocin!) and also encourages mum and baby bonding. The social aspect of these classes is so important too; sometimes all you need is a cup of tea and a chat.

Get some sleep. The sleep deprivation post baby is overwhelming. My son is now three and I still struggle with night waking and 5am starts. Ask your partner, mum, friend, anyone who can help to sit with baby for a couple of hours to allow you to catch up on your sleep. You are still a very important person and need to be rested and well to look after your new baby so catch some zeds when they are on offer.

The main thing is not make yourself feel worse by seeing yourself as weak or as an inadequate parent because you feel low. The fact that you care shows that you are a fantastic mum that's having a hard time. Every mum has been there, so please just reach out and speak to someone.

Moving towards a Rocking Birth and Baby

I hope you have enjoyed reading this book and don't feel like abandoning the whole idea of having a baby. I want to give you a quick summary of the things we've talked about to help you move towards your amazing, unique birth and gorgeous baby.

- Birth ROCKS. Look forward to birth with excitement, it's the most amazing thing you will ever do!
- Be honest with yourself and the people around you. What do you want? What do you need?
- Understand yourself. Peel back the layers, what really works for you? What comforts you?

- Look fear in the face. What are you scared of? How can you get rid of these fears? Who can help you do this?
- Try out different comfort techniques. Understand what is likely to comfort you during birth based on what comforts you in everyday life.
- Make a plan and be prepared not to stick to it. Have birth preferences and make the best choices for you and your baby, but be prepared to accept medical help if you want or need it on the day,
- Acceptance. Accept and love your birth no matter what it looks like. Don't feel the need to justify your birth choices and ditch the birth guilt!
- Love your baby and yourself. Look after yourself and accept help when you need it. You may now be a mummy, but you are still you and deserve all of the respect and love in the world.

Birth ROCKS® birth preparation programme

Did you know that Birth ROCKS®?

Child Preparation that's as individual as you are...

YogaBellies Birth ROCKS® is our bespoke natural childbirth preparation programme created and customized for parents to be. We believe that the day you give birth is the most amazing day of your life and we want to help you throughout your birthing experience.

One size does NOT fit all.

Birth ROCKS® does not teach 'one special technique' but instead promises to understand you and your birth partner and resultantly find the most positive birthing experience for you.

Our Mentors will work with you and your birth partner on a journey of self-discovery, releasing your fears of birth and understanding your own individual coping styles. We help you to create a custom birthing plan that works for YOU.

We will help you realise how amazing birth really is and allow you to just let it happen...

'Birth ROCKS' by Cheryl MacDonald is a complimentary resource to the Birth ROCKS® natural child birth preparation programme.

Aligning with the Birth ROCKS® philosophy this book aims to provide mothers-to-be and their partners with the support and guidance they need, helping to reduce their fears on the run up to their children's birth.

Rather than a formal 'how to' manual the book chooses not to instruct its readers but instead provides them with the knowledge they need to create a positive birthing experience. Just like the Birth ROCKS programme the book is a personal, supportive, and intimate portrait that also includes insights from a range of different women and their different childbirth experiences.

Reading Birth ROCKS enables women to realise that birth does not have to be frightening or painful and instead teaches its readers to believe that ultimately...

Birth ROCKS!

To find a mentor near you visit www.birthrocks.co.uk

Birth ROCKS® Your Questions Answered

What is the Birth ROCKS® programme?

An inspirational bespoke birth preparation course, customized to suit your birthing needs and coping preferences.

We don't promise you that one 'special technique' will work for everyone, what we do promise is to help you and your birth partner fully understand how you deal with new experiences and create a complete individual birthing experience for you, that will allow you to look forward to and enjoy the most amazing day of your life.

How are the sessions structured?

You will meet with your own Birth ROCKS® mentor before you begin your sessions to discuss your personal circumstances and what you hope to achieve from the sessions. This can be done in person or via phone or Skype. You have the option to attend small group sessions (no more than 5 couples) or to work with a Mentor on a one-to-one basis. You can attend an intensive one or two day workshop or you can space your sessions over 4 weeks. Just like your birth plan, the structure of the course can be adapted to meet the needs of you and your partner.

After the birth of your child, you will meet with your mentor again to discuss how your birth went and to conclude your 'journey' with your mentor.

What are the sessions like?

The sessions are informal and friendly, we won't be throwing around forceps or other scary medical toys and we won't be trying to scare you with horror stories or interventions. The purpose of Birth ROCKS® is to give you accurate and useful information and tools for birthing that will work for you.

The sessions involve group discussion, active participation in activities to prepare you for birth and 'homework' for you and your birth partner to continue your discussions of birth and parenting in between sessions. The sessions are fun, sometimes messy, sometimes emotional but always practical and useful.

Who is Birth ROCKS® for?

Birth ROCKS® is suitable for everyone, wither you are a first time mum or six time parent! We ask that you bring who you intend to be your birth partner on the day, so this could be your partner, husband, mum, friend or doula, it's up to you.

Birth ROCKS® was created with mum and her birth partner in mind. We don't run through a list of medical jargon and we won't waste your time with things you could read in books. We consider birth partner's role in the birth as much as mum herself and we focus on what the birth partner can do to support mum during the birth.

If I do Birth ROCKS®, will I have a pain free birth?

We're not going to lie to you, probably not :) Giving birth is hard work, but that doesn't mean it can't still be the most amazing experience of your life. We will help you approach birth with positivity and excitement and help you to minimize any discomfort you may experience. We are positive, but honest about birth and we won't make you any false promises.

Why do I need to prepare for birth?

You wouldn't turn up at a marathon without training, so why would you turn up birth without training? Nobody has to 'teach' you how to give birth; baby would come out if nobody was there. But we do need to prepare ourselves mentally and physically, by getting to know and understand ourselves, so that we can create the optimal circumstances for our individual birth.

If we go into birth with inaccurate or no information, then we are leaving ourselves at the mercy of medical staff.

What's Included?

Your Birth ROCKS® experience will include working from pregnancy to post birth with your own fully qualified Birth ROCKS® Mentor.

Our Birth ROCKS® mentors believe that One Size does NOT fit all when it comes to birth, and they will help you understand yourself and offer you comfort techniques and skills for birth to suit you as an individual.

A bit about YogaBellies®

What is YogaBellies®?

YogaBellies is yoga franchise that offers a range of pre and post natal classes and workshops in yoga for pregnancy and birth, for post-partum mum and baby, as well as baby massage and now also, yoga for children.

YogaBellies has quickly grown across the world and now offers like-minded individuals the opportunity to run their own YogaBellies classes and work around their family.

YogaBellies provide a range of unique classes for women and children of all ages.

YogaBellies® for Pregnancy

YogaBellies® for Pregnancy classes are gentle and safe for all women, whether new to Yoga or with years of practice with each week focusing on a different aspect of pregnancy and birth. This is more than just a yoga class, but also training in deep relaxation and preparation for birth and motherhood. We practise yoga postures suitable for pregnancy and birth, adjusted for each trimester; invaluable breathing techniques for pregnancy and labour and also relaxation and meditation techniques that mum can also use once baby arrives.

YogaBellies® for Mum & Baby

YogaBellies® Mum & Baby Yoga classes involve both mum and baby. A typical class includes baby stretches to take small bodies through a full range of movement which often astonishes and inspires their mummies including incorporating baby massage; breathing and focused yoga postures for the mums, and postures-for-two to give mums and babies new ways to relate to each other. For mummies, we focus on gently working the abdominal muscles, slowly getting mummy back to pre-baby shape and helping to build strength, stamina and fitness.

YogaBellies® Loving Touch Baby Massage

YogaBellies® Loving Touch classes are for infants from newborn age until 'mobile'(which can be anywhere between 6 and 10 months). Classes involve learning tactile massage techniques and strokes to aid growth, soothing and bonding for you and baby.

The benefits of infant massage for your child include;

- Smoothes the transition from womb to the world
- Develops baby's first language: touch
- Teaching positive loving touch
- Develops a feeling of being loved, respected and secure
- Develops body, mind, awareness and coordination
- Can help to reduce the discomfort of colic, wind and constipation
- Helps to regulate and strengthen baby's digestive and respiratory systems and stimulate circulatory and nervous systems
- Promotes relaxation
- Can help to reduce 'fussiness' and improve quality of sleep

YogaBellies® Little Angels Yoga (Mummy and Toddler Yoga)

YogaBellies® Little Angels' classes are aimed at babies aged 18 to 36 months and allow caregivers and toddlers to continue the bonding process through yoga and dry massage routines. The classes incorporate elements of yoga, massage, movement and music and continue the mum and baby bonding process while encouraging baby to express their new found creativity and freedom of expression. The class includes yoga postures and dry massage strokes as well as stories, music, singing songs and rhymes and heuristic play. These elements together help baby's vital development.

YogaBellies®Kidz Yoga

YogaBellies®Kidz yoga takes children age 3-12 years on a fantastical journey through the universe! YogaBelliesKidz sessions are written in line with the UK National Curriculum for Excellence and can see children journey through space, dive deep in the depths of the ocean, meet the Romans, meet exotic jungle animals and much much more. The postures focus on the things that excite and trigger the imagination of today's children. By engaging children in this positive way, we encourage them to use their imagination, become independent, resilient and strong. Each of our Kidz postures is grounded in traditional yoga with all of the benefits that adults can expect to see during a yoga practice, but with a much more gentle and fun approach.

YogaBellies® Mummy Therapies

YogaBellies® Mummy Therapies offer a range of perinatal holistic therapies for mummies including:

- Pre and post-partum massage,
- Beauty treatments for mummy
- A specialist combination of holistic therapies such as reflexology and reiki.

Our therapists are trained specifically to work with pregnant and post-partum mummies and use a range of gorgeous products for their treatments. All of our therapists are professionally trained and accredited by The Guild of Beauty Therapists and the IPTI. Our therapists can travel to the comfort of your own home, just to make life that little bit easier.

YogaBelles®

YogaBelles® classes encompass women at any stage of their life. The aim of YogaBelles is about discovering who you are as an individual and as a woman. Each class focuses towards one of four elements which include;

- o YogaBelles YIN: Restorative Yin Yoga
- o YogaBelles YANG: Core Strength Yoga
- o YogaBelles CHAKRA: Chakra Balance Yoga
- o YogaBelles LUNAR: Lunar Flow Yoga

YogaBelles does not use male centric positions and instead focuses towards enhancing the woman's abilities, her natural grace and femininity.

Visit

www.yogabellies.co.uk

and

www.birthrocks.co.uk

to find out more about us.